TIMELESS BEAUTY

TIMELESS BEAUTY

Everything You Want and Need to Know about Cosmetic Surgery and Procedures

Dr. Julie Khanna and Dr. Sheetal Sapra

with Lynda D. Prouse

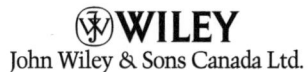

John Wiley & Sons Canada Ltd.

Copyright © 2004 by Dr. Julie Khanna, Dr. Sheetal Sapra, Lynda D. Prouse

All rights reserved. No part of this work covered by the copyright herein may be reproduced or used in any form or by any means—graphic, electronic or mechanical without the prior written permission of the publisher. Any request for photocopying, recording, taping or information storage and retrieval systems of any part of this book shall be directed in writing to The Canadian Copyright Licensing Agency (Access Copyright). For an Access Copyright license, visit www.accesscopyright.ca or call toll free 1-800-893-5777.

Care has been taken to trace ownership of copyright material contained in this book. The publisher will gladly receive any information that will enable them to rectify any reference or credit line in subsequent editions.

This publication contains the opinions and ideas of its author(s) and is designed to provide useful advice in regard to the subject matter covered. The author(s) and publisher are not engaged in rendering medical, therapeutic, or other services in this publication. This publication is not intended to provide a basis for action in particular circumstances without consideration by a competent professional. The author(s) and publisher expressly disclaim any responsibility for any liability, loss, or risk, personal or otherwise, which is incurred as a consequence, directly or indirectly, of the use and application of any of the contents of this book.

Library and Archives Canada Cataloguing in Publication

Prouse, Lynda,
    Timeless beauty : everything you want and need to know about cosmetic surgery and procedures / Julie Khanna, Sheetal Sapra, Lynda D. Prouse.

Includes index.
ISBN 0-470-83492-7

    1. Surgery, Plastic--Popular works.   I. Khanna, Julie   II. Sapra, Sheetal   III. Title.

RD119.P76 2004   617.9'52   C2004-906549-1

Production Credits:
Cover design: Sharon Foster Design
Interior text design: Mike Chan
Front cover photo: ©Elizabeth Knox/Masterfile

Printer: Transcontinental Printing

John Wiley & Sons Canada Ltd.
6045 Freemont Blvd.
Mississauga, Ontario
L5R 4J3

Printed in Canada

10 9 8 7 6 5 4 3 2 1

To our parents, who made us who we are, and to our children, Rahul and Deeya, for teaching us the meaning of true beauty.

Julie and Sheetal

To my mother Vera, and my sister Marlene, two of the most beautiful women I know, and in memory of my loving father, Bob, who always saw the beauty in me.

Lynda

CONTENTS

Acknowledgements	ix
Chapter 1: Mirror, Mirror on the Wall...	1
Chapter 2: All About Aging	9
Chapter 3: Nonablative Resurfacing of the Skin	29
Chapter 4: Medium and Deep Chemical Peels and Dermabrasion	53
Chapter 5: Laser Techniques	61
Chapter 6: Wrinkles	87
Chapter 7: Leg Veins	103
Chapter 8: Face, Brow, and Eye Lifts	109
Chapter 9: Facial Contouring	125
Chapter 10: Body Contouring	141
Chapter 11: Surgical Lifting for the Body	153
Chapter 12: Breast Enhancements	169
Chapter 13: Cosmetic Dentistry	187
Chapter 14: Hair Restoration	201
Chapter 15: Choosing a Qualified Specialist	211
Chapter 16: Preparing for Your Surgery	217
Index	223

ACKNOWLEDGEMENTS

The authors express their sincere gratitude to the following professionals for their generous contributions to this book:

Dr. Scott Powell, certified general surgeon for Chapter 7: Leg Veins; Dr. Issac Novak, cosmetic dentist for Chapter 13: Cosmetic Dentistry; and Dr. Vince Bertucci, cosmetic dermatologist for Chapter 14: Hair Restoration.

The authors would also like to thank:

The staff at the Institute of Cosmetic and Laser Surgery, and in particular, Karen Rosbrook and Brenda Dick.

Robert Harris and Don Loney at Wiley Publishers for believing in this book.

Joan Whitman at Wiley Publishing for her patience and editorial expertise, and also to project manager, Liz McCurdy and copy editor, Lisa Berland.

Arnold Gosewich for helping us to find a home for this book and looking after many of the details.

Lynda would also like to thank her husband David Szabo. Without his support, understanding, motivation and invaluable insight, this book and all of her previous books may not have been written.

In addition, Lynda thanks Julie and Sheetal for giving her the opportunity to write the book. Her respect for their integrity, honesty, knowledge and commitment to their patients is profound and she values their friendship.

Julie and Sheetal feel blessed to have each other for such a wonderful partnership in life and business. They would like to thank Lynda for helping to bring their vision to life. They believe this partnership has only been enhanced by Lynda's writing expertise and collaboration with her in the production of this book.

Last, but not least, Julie and Sheetal would like to thank their patients for motivating and trusting them to produce this book.

Chapter 1

Mirror, Mirror
on the Wall ...

Since the beginning of time, beauty has been sought and coveted as if it were the rarest of treasures. While Cleopatra probably welcomed the many exotic gifts and precious gems bestowed upon her by rulers of far-away kingdoms, history has shown she was equally fascinated in the ways women from other lands beautified themselves. Indeed, this ruler of ancient Egypt spent countless hours soaking in baths of milk and honey in an attempt to soften her skin, applied crushed stone to her body to exfoliate roughness, and went through a daily ritual in which various primitive cosmetics were painted on her face. All were done with a longing to look younger and more beautiful—a premise most modern women, who would love the sight of a flawless complexion reflecting back from their own mirrors, would understand.

Having skin that is free of wrinkles, sagging, and dullness has been important to the female sector throughout the ages, but as the majority of the North American population approaches and passes the half-century mark, the search for the all elusive fountain of youth has reached an almost feverish pitch. Americans alone spend over $12 billion a year on cosmetics to counteract aging. A peek into most women's vanity cupboards, where there will likely be an array of cosmetic treatments that would boggle the most serious of chemists' minds, would confirm this statistic. Toners, cleansers, pore minimizers, exfoliaters, topical vitamins and creams, serums, and lotions for the eyes, throat, décolleté, face, and body that claim to soften, erase wrinkles, rejuvenate, firm, and lift the skin are being created and sold to women, who are buying into the hype and promises of hope in a bottle.

Research indicates that 80 percent of all women are dissatisfied with some aspect of their appearance. They're watching the beauty infomercials on television and purchasing the products, reading the magazine articles touting the newest and best in anti-aging products and taking advantage of the numerous cosmetic procedures that are currently available. And it's not just women. Although most men would have a difficult time admitting it, the passing of the years and the havoc age plays on their bodies and faces does bother them. As their wives and partners appear to grow more youthful through cosmetic treatments with each birthday, men want to close the illusionary age gap. They also need to remain competitive at work. Ever since Bill Gates became the CEO of one of the world's largest companies, the entire outlook of who is in charge changed. If it's a man, the president of the company is no longer a grey-haired, grandfatherly figure. He's usually someone with an energetic, dynamic presence, often appearing to be in his thirties or forties. Although valuable, experience is taking second place to vibrancy. To stay in the game, whether a man or a woman, one must remain youthful and attractive in guise.

Our new reality television shows include extreme makeovers, beauty pageant plastic surgery that transforms "ugly ducklings" into swans, and entertainment programs featuring the secret cosmetic procedures of celebrities. We sit

Chapter 1| Mirror, Mirror on the Wall ...

mesmerized by the incredible alterations that take place before our eyes, and can't escape even during the commercials, which tell us what product to buy in order to appear younger and more beautiful. Even one of the top new television dramas revolves around the practice of two plastic surgeons and their clients.

Although most people are likely not considering an extreme makeover of their own, they may want to enhance or change at least one aspect of their appearance. Studies show that if we improve the way we look, we can often improve the way we feel. Our confidence grows and we're able to face the day with a more positive outlook. When we look and feel better, people treat us better, because in our society, appearance does matter.

According to social psychologists, from the time we were children and were read bedtime stories that spoke of the beautiful princess/handsome prince and the ugly witch/gruesome ogre, we subconsciously related good to beautiful and bad to ugly. Research on physical attraction finds this association carries on throughout our lives and affects the way we are treated and the way we treat others. Further studies indicate that a cuter baby is given more affection than a homely baby, and the more attractive children are, the better grades they will receive in school. A good-looking adult will usually get the better job, higher salary, and more recognition. They are perceived as being successful, intelligent, personable, and competent. One U.S. study even suggested that taller men were paid $600 more per inch than shorter men. These same studies conclude that less attractive people often struggle through their careers and relationships.

Based on this data, it would seem that a better-looking human being will have higher self-esteem from an early age, based on the way he or she was treated from infancy onward. The theory that beautiful is good, and ugly is bad, becomes a self-fulfilling prophecy. Sad but true. And as we grow older and lose the bloom of youth, Western society in particular has deemed that aging is unattractive. So no matter if we were good-looking when we were thirty. At sixty, we're considered "over-the-hill." With our life expectancy dramatically increasing over the last several decades, this does not bode well for the baby boomers, who through diet, exercise, and modern medicine are much healthier than their grandparents were at the same age. They want to look as good on the outside as they feel on the inside.

In generations past, if one was lucky enough to reach the "golden years," aging of the skin—which includes wrinkles, furrows, bags, hanging jowls, discolorations, growths, sagging, and dryness—was thought of as nothing more than the price you had to pay for living a longer life. But it is something we no longer have to accept. Whereas, in days gone by, our predecessors may have believed a facelift was frivolous, vain, time-consuming, and expensive, with the new noninvasive cosmetic procedures now available, we can take years off our faces during lunch hour. Techniques such as Botox, Restylane, Artecoll, collagen, and fat injections that treat facial lines and wrinkles are fast becoming a habitual part of many adult lives. In fact, many woman consider Botox to be a part of their regular beauty routine. And why not? Instead of spending our money on cosmetic creams that seldom deliver the goods they promise, a few injections of Botox can help erase the ravages of time quickly and with little or no pain.

Certain laser procedures, which produce a smoother, younger skin, have lasting results and can give us a more youthful, radiant look, while other laser techniques effectively rid the skin of unwanted blemishes, age or sun spots, facial blood vessels, tattoos, and scars. Other quick and noninvasive beauty procedures include chemical peels, microdermabrasion, photo facials (IPL), thermoplastic contouring, laser hair removal, and leg vein treatments.

Cosmetic surgery is also on the rise, with face, brow, and eyelid lifts being performed on a daily basis in North

America. Nose reshaping, lip augmentation, and chin and cheek contouring are all popular aesthetic procedures, as are techniques that make it possible to reshape the breasts, abdomen, thighs, and other parts of the body.

According to the American Society for Aesthetic Plastic Surgery, the overall number of cosmetic procedures (both surgical and nonsurgical) has increased 228 percent since 1997. In 2003, approximately 8.3 million procedures were done in the United States, with Americans spending just under $9.4 billion on cosmetic procedures. Botox injections made up close to three million of those procedures, while chemical peels and microdermabrasion accounted for just under a million each. Hundreds of thousands of other Americans underwent nose reshaping, liposuction, breast enhancement, eyelid surgery, and facelifts. In Canada, over $500 million was spent on cosmetic procedures in 2003, says the Rotman School of Business at the University of Toronto, with over 100,000 Botox injections being given. That same year also saw a 52 percent rise in facelifts and 17 percent more breast augmentations, with liposuction following close behind.

This is an industry that doctors Sheetal Sapra and Julie Khanna, husband and wife and partners at the Institute of Cosmetic and Laser Surgery, know well. Dr. Sapra is a Fellow of the Royal College of Physicians of Canada and the American Academy of Dermatology, and is also a diplomate of the American Board of Dermatology, a member of the Canadian Dermatology Association, the Canadian Laser Aesthetics Surgery Society, American Society of Dermatological Surgery, the International Society of Dermatological Surgery, the American Society for Laser Medicine and Surgery, the American Contact Dermatitis Society, and the Toronto and Ottawa Dermatological Society. An attending dermatologist at the Oakville Trafalgar Memorial Hospital, prior to opening his private practice, Dr. Sapra was an assistant professor at Queens University and is currently an advisor, educator, and spokesperson for laser products and various injectables, such as Botox and Restylane.

Dr. Julie Khanna is an attending plastic surgeon at the Oakville Trafalgar Memorial Hospital, and is certified by the Royal College of Physicians and Surgeons of Canada and a diplomate of the American Board of Plastic Surgeons. She is also a member of the Canadian Society of Plastic Surgeons, Canadian Society for Aesthetic Plastic Surgery, the American Society for Aesthetic Plastic Surgery, the American Society of Plastic Surgeons and the American Society for Laser Medicine and Surgery. Dr. Khanna also does volunteer work worldwide with nonprofit organizations that help children with facial deformities. Both the doctors regularly appear on television and radio programs that educate the public on the pros and cons of cosmetic procedures and surgery.

Although doctors Sapra and Khanna still see patients for medical concerns, they found that in the past few years, there has been an increasing surge towards noninvasive cosmetic treatments. According to Dr. Sapra, and the American Society for Aesthetic Plastic Surgery, while plastic cosmetic surgery such as breast enhancement, liposuction, and tummy tucks are becoming increasingly popular, the biggest growth rate is in the nonsurgical procedures, which include Botox, fillers, nonablative lasers, photo facials, photo rejuvenation, non-surgical facelifts, and nonsurgical dissolving of fat in the skin. There has also been a tremendous upswing in mild chemical peels and microdermabrasion. These techniques can slowly turn back the clock by five to six years without dramatic change or an artificial appearance to the face. Dr. Sapra says this trend began in the early 1990s, when light chemical peels, power peels, and collagen fillers were developed.

Adding to the interest was the advancement in lasers such as the carbon dioxide laser, which targets wrinkles and which may result in less downtime than surgical procedures such as a facelift. During this period, an understanding of what causes aging came to the forefront, and the prevention and treatment soon followed, with products such as Retin-A, Renova, and alpha hydroxy acids being introduced.

In a few short years, it was realized that something could be done about aging that didn't involve a drastic and costly procedure that would often take months to heal. Women went for it in a big way.

But according to Dr. Khanna, the popularity in cosmetic and surgical procedures has also taken place because altering one's appearance has become more acceptable than it was in the past. She theorizes there has been an empowerment of women, who believe they have the right to make decisions and change their lives if they wish to. This general empowerment, which began with the right to vote then moved on to allow women to earn their own money and eventually gave them the freedom to have children without a partner, is what now gives women permission to make their own choices about the way they look. If a woman doesn't like something about herself, she doesn't have to accept it. There are options available and the contemporary woman is free to explore them.

What Dr. Khanna finds just as interesting is the changing attitude in men towards their own appearance. Traditionally, it is not as common for this gender to change as it is for women. In days gone by, men rarely altered their hair colour, hair style, or clothing, and tended not to be victims of fashion and trends like their female counterparts. However, now that society—and to be more specific, their male peers—has recently deemed it okay for even the most macho to modify or improve his appearance, men are taking advantage of various cosmetic treatments, with hair restoration being their favourite, followed by Botox and liposuction.

Even though cosmetic alterations of the face and body are definitely the wave of the future, Drs. Sapra and Khanna are quick to point out the various techniques are not for everyone. Indeed, both doctors will often turn away patients with unrealistic expectations. For example, if someone with deep pockmark scars believed that microdermabrasion would dramatically smooth their skin, he or she would have to be refused, as would be those who wanted a too tiny nose that would be totally out of proportion with the rest of their face. Age can often play a part in these rejections. Dr. Khanna will not operate on anyone until they have fully developed into adulthood, unless the circumstances are extreme or medically related, while Dr. Sapra has to often turn down older women, who believe a chemical peel will magically erase their decades' worth of wrinkles.

This book, a collaboration between the doctors and author Lynda D. Prouse, explores most, if not all, areas of cosmetic surgery, techniques, and treatments, including the many myths and misconceptions that surround the topic. Our ultimate goal is to offer the most complete, honest, and comprehensive guide to cosmetic procedures, from Botox to breast enhancements and then some. We will tell you what works and what doesn't and what any given procedure can or cannot do. We describe the technique or operation and its background, let you know how much downtime is involved, what the complications and risks can be, any post-treatment that may be required, whether and when the procedure will have to be repeated, how much it all approximately costs, and whether or not any given technique is for you. Our aim is to educate regarding the entire spectrum of choices available in cosmetic procedures and surgery, and give you the information and understanding you require to weigh the pros and cons and then make an informed decision.

By the way, don't throw out your cosmetic creams and lotions just yet because, as you'll soon discover, depending on the ingredients, some of them actually do provide results! But we'll discuss that soon enough. For now, let's turn the page and find out what causes aging and what we can do about it.

Chapter 2

All About Aging

The moment we are born our skin begins to age. Occurring throughout our entire body as we grow older, this is referred to as *intrinsic* aging, meaning it is caused by internal factors. Essentially, this type of aging is genetically programmed, and these genetics are different for each and every person. Every facial expression we make is also genetically preprogrammed—we only have to look at our parents or grandparents to foresee what we'll most likely look like at their age. And since we make countless numbers of facial expressions throughout our lifetime, the corresponding muscles are used on a habitual basis. Up until about age twenty, these expressions have little effect on our appearance. But as we grow older our skin gets thinner and, over time, the underlying network of elastin and collagen, which supports the structure of the skin, becomes more fragile, resulting in a loss of elasticity. The skin then begins to sag and form lines and furrows. It becomes drier, loses its glow, and doesn't bounce back like it did in our youth.

Although no one person can say with definitive proof why intrinsic aging occurs in the body, it is generally theorized that free radicals play a huge part. Although difficult to describe in a generalized term, a free radical is basically an unstable oxygen molecule generated by chemical reactions that occur in the body. This unstable oxygen species reacts and interacts with other cells and molecules around it, causing damage to healthy skin cells in the epidermis and dermis. Even though our bodies have internal systems, called antioxidants, that quench free radicals, as we age we lose the ability to quell or completely eliminate them. The free radicals eventually overwhelm the body's antioxidant system and the skin becomes more and more damaged.

The other cause of aging is called *extrinsic,* meaning it is caused by external factors. This type of aging is mainly caused by sun exposure, smoking, air pollution or other environmental toxins, poor nutrition or diets that are not rich in antioxidants (vitamins and minerals), excess alcohol consumption, and stress. All of the above will accelerate the aging process, but by far the worst offender is the sun.

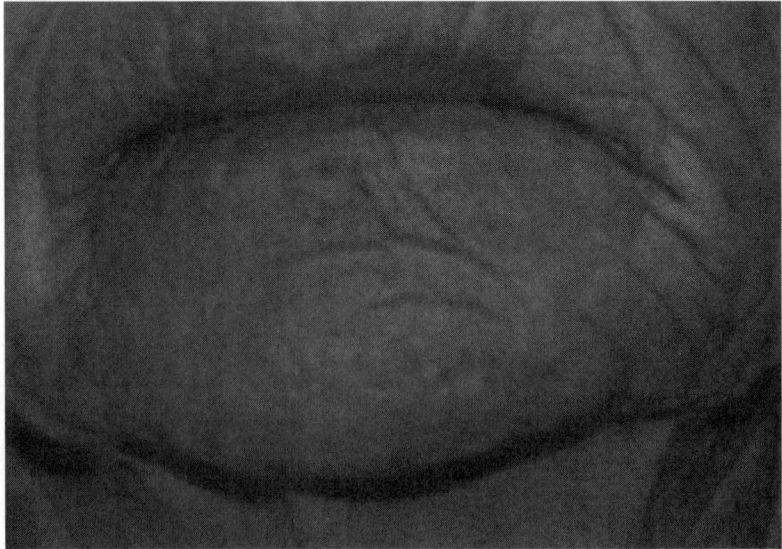

Facial aging wrinkles.

Chapter 2| **All About Aging** 11

Labelled "photo-aging," sun damage through excessive exposure to ultraviolet "A" (UVA) and ultraviolet "B" (UVB) rays is the most common cause of extrinsic aging. When these harmful rays of sunlight hit the body, they increase the generation of free radicals, which in turn ravage the skin. The damage begins the moment we go into the sun and becomes more evident as time goes on. Causing dramatic changes to occur, exposure to UVA and UVB rays will prompt the skin to become drier and thinner. Increased and irregular pigmentation will develop, showing up in a yellowing of the overall skin, brown spots (called lentigo) that are also referred to as "age spots," and broken blood vessels. Wrinkles begin to develop more quickly than they would through the natural aging process, and eventually become very deep as the skin takes on a weathered, leathery look.

If any woman wants to see what photo-aging does to the skin, she should stand in front of a mirror undressed and look at the area directly under her breasts. Most likely this area will be clear and creamy white if she is Caucasian, and lighter than the surrounding area if she is a woman with a

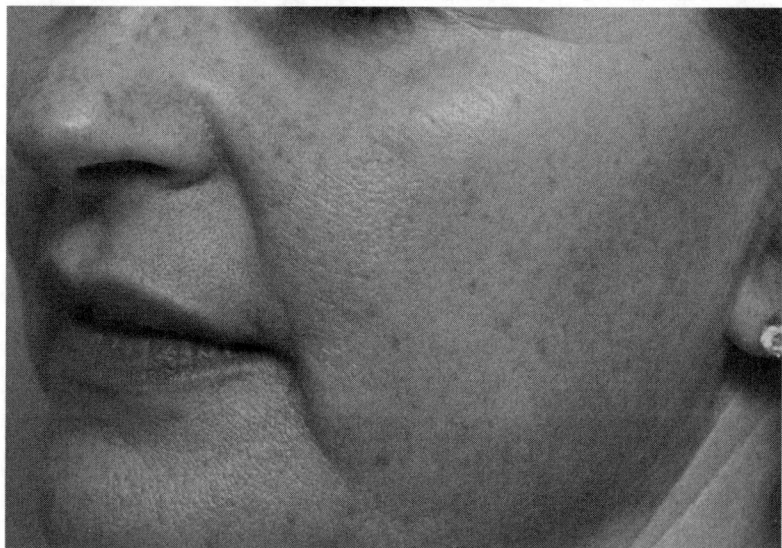

Sun damage.

darker complexion. Then she only has to compare the usually hidden breast area with her chest and face, where wrinkles, brown spots, broken blood vessels, and a wide array of other skin imperfections will be visibly noticeable. Most, if not all, of the damage is caused by the sun. Doctors will often classify the level of damage caused by photo-aging using the following system called the "Glogau Classification", which has been simplified for the purpose of this book.

Glogau Classification

Damage	Characteristics	Description
Type 1 (mild)	"No wrinkles"	Early photo-aging • Ages 20–30 • Mild pigment changes • No keratoses (abnormal cells) • minimal wrinkles
Type 2 (moderate)	"Wrinkles in motion" Early to moderate photo-aging	• Wrinkles starting to form • Age: late thirties to forties • Some pigment changes • Keratoses apparent but not visible • Parallel smile lines appear

Type 3 (advanced)	"Wrinkles at rest" Advanced photo-aging	• Wrinkles present when not moving • Age: fifties • Visible pigment changes • Visible keratoses • wrinkles present when not moving
Type 4 (severe)	"Only wrinkles" Severe photo-aging	• Age: sixties and older • Yellow-grey skin colour • Prior skin malignancies • No normal skin

Although our skin type, which is outlined in the chart below, predisposes us to photo-aging and will distinguish the type of aging process that will happen, this damage will most definitely occur in one form or another to anyone who is overexposed to the sun. In fact, apart from accelerating the aging process, overexposure may further cause grave medical harm, including various forms of skin cancer. There is absolutely no way to get around it: other than a cosmetic-type tanning solution or bronzer, there is no such thing as a "safe tan." And this includes tanning beds, where the ultraviolet rays are just as devastating to the skin as the sun.

Generally, skin can be classified into these six different types:

Fitzpatrick Skin Type Classification

Skin Type	Skin Colour	Characteristics
1	White	Burns, never tans
2	White	Burns and sometimes tans
3	White	Mildly burns and also tans
4	White	Seldom burns, tans more than average
5	Brown	Seldom burns, tans deeply
6	Black	Never burns

Usually the lighter the skin, the more likelihood there will be of pigmentation change, broken blood vessels and wrinkling from sun damage. With darker skin tones, especially in skin types 5 and 6, the chance of permanent pigmentation change and sun damage is decreased.

Because we can't escape from the sun, and indeed, sunlight is necessary to all of us to promote a general feeling of well-being and provide vitamin D to our bodies, it is advised to wear a sun protection factor (SPF) containing titanium dioxide and/or zinc oxide of at least 15 every day throughout the year on any parts of our body that are not covered by clothing, whether or not we are in direct sunlight. Premature wrinkling and damage to our skin can occur while sitting in the shade in the summer, walking the dog in the snow, or even in the car at any time of the year during our daily commutes back and forth to work. Hats are back in fashion, and wearing one can only bring further protection to your face. If you must overexpose yourself to the sun, try not to do it in the peak hours between 11:00 a.m. and 4:00 p.m., and wear a sunscreen of 30 or higher. And remember, most sunscreens are not waterproof. If you're swimming or perspiring, reapply the protection often.

Other than staying out of the sun and applying an appropriate sunscreen daily, there are other ways that we can prevent the effects of aging from showing up on our skin. While cosmetics can help to make the skin appear to be younger, smoother, firmer, and less wrinkled, they are temporary in what they do and will not cause a long-lasting change to the skin itself. Most cosmetics work in one of three ways. They will either hydrate or moisturize, blocking the release of water from the skin so it plumps up and feels better to the touch. Others will produce a low-grade inflammation, which causes the skin to swell, temporarily removing the fine lines and wrinkles. Lastly, cosmetics will cover up the imperfections, either through colour, such as foundations, powders, and concealers, or through silicone-type gels that transiently blur the fine lines. Unfortunately, once all of these varieties of cosmetics are washed off, the flaws become noticeable once again.

Use cosmetics for what they are intended—to make your skin look and feel better, but just be aware few will help to make any permanent changes in your skin. A perfect analogy would be to look at cosmetics and what they can do for your skin in the same way that you look at shampoo and what it can do for your hair. If we don't shampoo our hair regularly, it doesn't look good and can affect the way we feel about ourselves. When we wash our hair, it becomes soft, shiny, and easier to manage, and we feel great. There isn't an actual change to our hair, only in its appearance. Cosmetics work in much the same way. They may help us to look and feel good on a temporary basis, but few will have any significant or long-term effects on our skin. Wonderful cosmetics that serve just this purpose are available, and they have a definite and important part to play in the way we feel about ourselves, but they are not a magic elixir for preventing and removing wrinkles or firming up sagging skin. If they were so miraculous, there wouldn't be any old-looking people in the world.

To re-emphasize, the most important "cosmetic" that anyone can use is a sunscreen with an SPF of 15 or higher. If you want to incorporate a moisturizer in your daily routine (although most sunscreens are moisturizers in that they hydrate the skin by their emollient consistency), ensure the ingredients of the cream or lotion include a sun protection factor.

Because the skin on your face is different and usually more delicate than the skin on your body, you should use a different type of moisturizer on the face than on the body. Again, make certain the moisturizer you use on your body contains a sunscreen. But as far as purchasing different creams for various parts of the face (eye, neck, mouth) or the body (décolleté, hands, feet, thighs), it really is unnecessary and a waste of money. A cream that works well on your hands will work equally well on your feet. And the same applies to the different parts of your face. Other than the eyelid area, which for most people is extremely sensitive and can often react to the most mild of creams, if a product causes irritation when you put it under your eyes, it probably shouldn't be used on the rest of your face either. Stinging eyes are the first sign that your body is reacting to a foreign substance that it doesn't agree with. And if you are using an eye cream and are noticing a reduction in fine lines and wrinkles, the product is probably causing some swelling. Your wrinkles disappear for a few hours because of the inflammation, but the cream is certainly not getting rid of them.

A good moisturizer contains emollients and other agents that help to keep water in the skin, but most also contain a myriad of other ingredients that, when applied in layers (using several creams instead of one), can be irritating or even harmful to the skin. And if you have oily skin, you should avoid using moisturizers altogether. They encourage blackheads by clogging the pores, cause the skin to become dull as dead skin cells adhere in the oils and hair follicles, and can even bring on outbreaks of dermatitis and other skin ailments. Like life, the key to good skin care is to keep it simple.

Having said all this about cosmetics, there are a handful of topical substances that can be applied to the skin, which have shown to assist in the prevention and treatment of wrinkles. The following are the most important.

VITAMIN A/TRETINOIN

Tretinoin is the acid form of vitamin A or retinol, scientifically referred to as all-trans retinoic acid, which is important for skin health. Commonly known by brand names Retin-A or Renova, it was originally and still is used to treat acne and is the only topical agent proven to treat photo-aging. Tretinoin is currently available through a doctor's prescription.

Using tretinoin on a regular basis for a period of approximately four to six months will assist in rebuilding collagen and elastin, smoothing out the skin's texture and making it thicker and plumper while decreasing the size of wrinkles. An added benefit is the glow that tretinoin puts back into the skin and the lightening and removal of some of the pigmentation changes such as freckles and brown spots. However, tretinoin can be irritating, causing some peeling, dryness, and redness, and not all skin types can tolerate the treatment.

Formulated in four strengths of concentration (0.01%, 0.025%, .05% and 0.1%), tretinoin should be applied beginning with the lowest strength. Using a pea-sized amount, smooth the cream over the face, every third or fourth night initially before building up to nightly for a few months. Then you may move up to the next level of concentration. When the highest strength is reached, the program should be maintained by applying the cream every few days. Although the eyelid area should be avoided, once the skin has adapted to the cream a small amount can be dabbed under the eyes, where many have noticed an improvement in the appearance of fine lines with continued use. However, because tretinoin is a form of acid, and the eye area can be more delicate in some individuals, the diminishment in fine lines may be due to a low-grade inflammation and subsequent swelling.

Tretinoin should only be applied at night since wearing it in sunlight may actually cause the skin to burn. People who can tolerate the side effects of tretinoin can begin treatment in their twenties, or whenever they notice the first signs of sun damage, and continue using it for the rest of their lives. However, pregnant woman should avoid the use of tretinoin.

It must be remembered that the effects of tretinoin are very different from retinol's. Many cosmetic companies are loading their products with retinol or a milder form of vitamin A called retinyl palmitate, and claiming it to be as potent as Retin-A or Renova, without the irritation or the doctor's prescription. But the amount of retinol or retinyl palmitate would have to be extremely high on the product's ingredient list to have any benefit whatsoever. And even then, because vitamin A is an unstable molecule, there is no way of knowing whether or not the type put into the cosmetic formulation would be active on the skin. One tell-tale sign that the vitamin A in a product is at least purporting to be

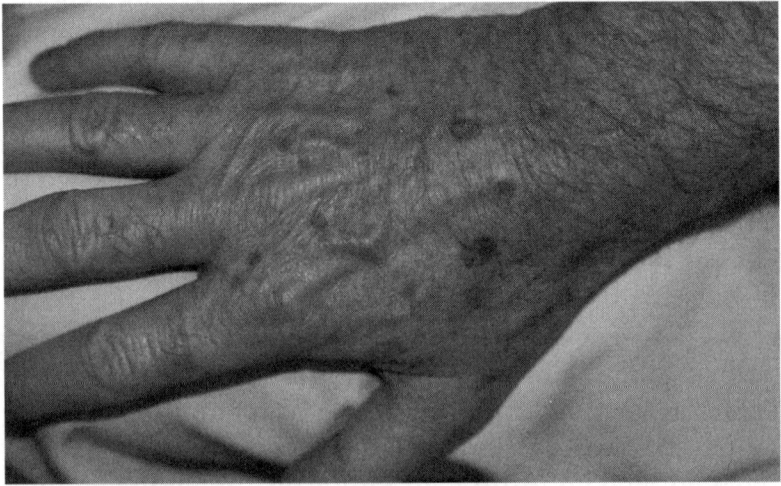

Age spots on the hands.

stable is the type of packaging the cosmetic comes in, because the vitamin will begin to deteriorate once exposed to light and air. Both Renova and Retin-A are housed in metallic-like tubes that are safety sealed and airtight. The bottle, jar, or tube containing the retinol or retinyl palmitate must be opaque, and this applies to all other topically applied antioxidants that will be discussed in this chapter.

VITAMIN C

Vitamin C or L-ascorbic acid (a form of vitamin C) is an antioxidant that, added onto our own body's antioxidant system, helps to squelch the free radicals on our skin. When applied topically, it helps to diminish fine lines and wrinkles and adds a radiant clarity to the skin tone, making it brighter and appear more youthful. Applied in the morning directly onto the skin before any moisturizers, toners, or other cosmetics, vitamin C may also protect the skin from sun damage. However, this protection is only limited to UVA rays, so it does not take the place of a sunscreen.

The only downside to vitamin C is that this particular vitamin is probably one of the most unstable antioxidants, so it will immediately break down or oxidize upon exposure to light and air. Some cosmetic companies profess that by enclosing the vitamin C in an individual capsule, powdered form, opaque tube or brown bottle, the vitamin will remain active. However, aside from the type of packaging the vitamin is housed in, it is difficult to know whether or not the product was stabilized in the first place. The most stable form of this vitamin would be a vitamin C ester, which is a derivative of the original vitamin. But as with all products, it is wise to try different formats of vitamin C and see what works best for you, keeping in mind that it will do you no good if it is not listed at the top of an ingredient list (meaning it is the main ingredient), identified as active and stable, and housed in the proper packaging. It should also contain a concentration of at least 10 percent to be of any effect.

VITAMIN E

There are several forms of vitamin E, but it is the alpha tocopherol, tocotrienol, and tocopherol acetate formations that are believed to be particularly beneficial to the skin when applied topically. Thought to slow the signs of aging, vitamin E is also known for its proprieties that help to reverse cell damage caused by persistent exposure to the sun. Specifically, it is believed to hydrate, reduce the size of wrinkles, and improve the overall texture of the skin. Like its potent cousin, vitamin C, it also provides some measure of protection from UVA rays, but again, it is not a substitute for a sunscreen.

ALPHA HYDROXY ACIDS (AHAs)

Although several types of alpha hydroxy acids are being sold in the marketplace, only glycolic acid and lactic acid are of particular benefit because they are able to penetrate the skin's surface and help to regenerate our collagen and elastin. With a sugarcane base, glycolic acid is undoubtedly the most important of the two chemicals since it is able to penetrate the skin more readily than lactic acid, which has a base of sour milk and has a larger molecular structure. However, both acids were touted as miracle solutions for many years with claims that by simply rubbing them on your skin, it would become wrinkle-free. This was and is untrue. Used at high strengths they will only peel the outer surface of the skin, remove dead skin cells, encourage new cell production, unclog the pores, and reduce some fine wrinkling. The use of glycolic acid will also lighten some pigmentation changes caused by sun damage. After treatment of either of the acids, the skin will feel softer and smoother with a noticeable improvement in the appearance of fine lines and the overall texture of the skin. Because dead skin cells often cause the skin to take on a greyish and dull cast, without them adhering to the face the skin will be rosier. Moisturizers will be more easily absorbed, which in turn hydrate the face and temporarily plump it up.

Chapter 2| All About Aging

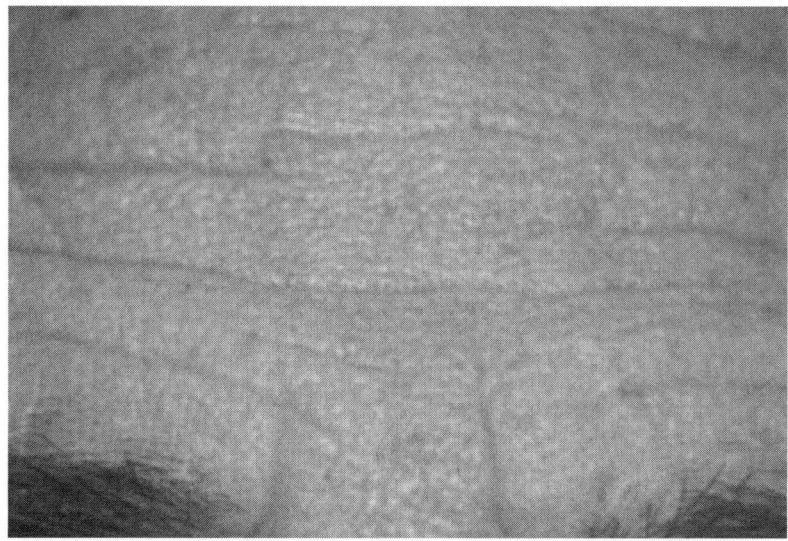
Facial aging of brow.

In order for an alpha hydroxy to be of any benefit, it should be used at a strength of 8 to 10 percent and must have a pH of 3 to 4. While there are cosmetics in the marketplace that do contain these amounts, most only consist of about 3 to 6 percent of the acids, and few list the pH value, making it difficult to determine the effectiveness of the product.

It must be cautioned that very high levels of the acids (12 plus), should only be used under the supervision of a dermatologist. Because the use of an alpha hydroxy acid can increase susceptibility to damage from the sun's rays, it should be applied at night. If your face is not overly sensitive to the product, you can use the acids on a prolonged basis. Always avoid the eyelid area and use on just-cleansed skin before applying a moisturizer.

BETA HYDROXY ACIDS (BHAs)

Beta hydroxy or salicylic acids have much of the same properties as AHAs, with the main difference between them being that the BHAs are oil-soluble while AHAs are water-soluble. Because of this, BHAs have the ability to infiltrate the oil in the pores and remove dead skin cells from the oil gland, which is particularly beneficial to those suffering from blackheads and other debris in the pores.

The following information is the sole opinion of the authors, based on our experience, both personal and with patients, at the time of this writing. It is not based on any clinical trials that we have performed.

Now that we have determined what can work topically on the skin, let's examine some of the latest buzzwords coming from the cosmetic industry. According to advertisements, these so-called miracle ingredients will do everything from removing wrinkles to firming up sagging skin. Some claim that you will see up to ten years erased from your face. Following are some of the more talked-about ingredients and what we believe they really do.

Argireline (aka Arjerolin)
Claims: Will work on the skin topically to remove wrinkles, especially around the eyes and the brow, and is almost as effective as Botox injections in relaxing the muscles.
Fact: A synthetic peptide, Argireline is an active ingredient in some creams and is fairly new. We have found little substantiated evidence to support the claim that it will relax the muscles. It would appear that this is just another good moisturizer.

Aloe Vera
Claims: Heals the skin and smooths wrinkles.
Fact: The juice from the aloe vera plant does have an anti-irritant effect when applied to the skin directly from the plant. However, like many other natural products, aloe juice is unstable, and any healing components will deteriorate when removed from the source. Unless processed in a certain and exacting manner, it will be of little benefit in healing the skin. Even if aloe juice is immediately applied from a plant to the skin, it will not get rid of wrinkles.

Alpha Lipoic Acid

Claims: When it is introduced to the skin, it will enter the cells and provide protection from free radical damage and dramatically improve aging skin.

Fact: Like vitamins C and E, research indicates this may be a good antioxidant when applied topically to the skin, and as such, may also help to improve skin tone and texture.

Amino Acids

Claims: Improves the look and texture of the skin.

Fact: Amino acids are found in various forms of animal and plant proteins. When put into a skin cream, they may act as an emollient but will otherwise have little effect on the skin.

Coenzyme Q10 (Ubiquinone)

Claims: Reduces wrinkles.

Fact: While coenzyme Q10 is a nutrient, and does have some internal antioxidant properties, we don't believe that it has much effect on the skin when applied topically.

Collagen

Claims: By adding collagen to a cosmetic, it will help regenerate the collagen in the body, causing a more youthful look.

Fact: It is difficult for collagen that has been taken from animals or plants to penetrate the skin. Even if it did, collagen fibres added to cosmetics will not rebuild the body's natural collagen and will have little effect on improving wrinkles or sagging skin.

Copper

Claims: Erases wrinkles, protects the skin and helps repair it.

Fact: While important for human nutrition and effective in healing wounds, copper has not been proven to be of much benefit in erasing wrinkles when applied topically.

DMAE (Dimethylaminoethanol)

Claims: Improves wrinkles and has skin firming and lifting benefits.

Fact: Some experts believe that when DMAE is taken orally, it may improve physical performance. However, there is little evidence that when applied to the skin it will have much benefit.

Elastin

Claims: By adding elastin to the cosmetic and applying it to the skin, it will assist in rebuilding natural elastin, culminating in a more youthful appearance.

Fact: Topically applied elastin will have no effect on regenerating the body's own elastin.

Grape Seed Extract

Claims: Improves the texture of the skin and evens out pigmentation.

Fact: Containing the powerful antioxidant proanthocyanidin, grape seed extract is good for the body when taken orally. However, we have found little evidence that it is beneficial to the skin when applied topically. When grape seed oil is mixed with pure vitamin E, there are some skin softening properties, as there are in most oils.

Green Tea

Claims: Has a healing effect on the skin.

Fact: There is data showing that green tea (and black tea) is an excellent antioxidant when taken internally, but we don't believe that it has much healing effect on the skin when applied topically.

Hyaluronic Acid

Claims: Is an excellent moisturizer that will rejuvenate the skin.

Fact: Although a satisfactory water-binding agent, (which is important in the making of an adequate moisturizer), unless formulated in a very small molecular structure, hyaluronic acid is unable to penetrate the skin unless injected as a filler. When applied topically, it is a good moisturizer, but does little else in improving the appearance of the skin.

Matrixil
Claims: Rebuilds collagen.
Fact: Little data could be found on this ingredient, other than that it supposedly contains a chain of amino acids (which are proteins) and peptides. However, other than alpha and beta hydroxy acids, tretinoin and dermatologist treatments, we know of no cosmetic ingredient that can rebuild the body's natural collagen.

Olive Oil
Claims: Has effective anti-aging properties when applied to the skin.
Fact: Olive oil used for cooking is a good antioxidant when taken internally, but other than its excellent moisturizing abilities, it will do little else for the skin when applied topically. Some forms of skin creams and oils, containing high amounts of first-pressed olive oil, seem to have soothing effects, as well as excellent emollient properties, but this could be due to the other ingredients added to the products.

Oglio-Peptide
Claims: Works better than retinol or vitamin C in thickening the skin, reducing wrinkles and skin roughness.
Facts: Found in a popular stretch mark cream, oglio-peptide cannot penetrate the skin and it is unlikely that it would have much effect on wrinkles, other than softening them with the moisturizing properties that would be included in the original stretch mark formulation.

Peptides
Claims: Thickens the skin over a three to six month period.
Facts: A peptide is a form of protein, which can have emollient properties to soften the skin, but it cannot penetrate, thus having no effect on the density of the skin.

Soy
Claims: Improves skin tone and texture.
Facts: Soybeans are a natural form of protein, and when used in cosmetics, may have skin-softening properties, thus improving the tone and texture by temporarily plumping the skin.

Torricelum
Claims: Moisturizes, reduces wrinkles, firms and tones skin.
Facts: Other than alluding that torricelum is taken from the sea, the company that manufactures this ingredient does not say what it is composed of. However, it appears to be an exceptional moisturizer and does improve the tone of the skin and the appearance of fine lines and wrinkles through its moisturizing properties, which temporarily plump the skin.

Vitamin K
Claims: Reduces the appearance of dark circles under the eyes and constricts capillaries.
Facts: Only studies prepared by those with an interest in selling vitamin K products are available; we know of no unbiased research done to prove these claims to be true.

Cosmeceuticals/Physicians' Cosmetic Products
Claims: Denoting a medical association, a "cosmeceutical" product combines pharmaceutical and dermatological properties and is therefore better for the skin.

Chapter 2| **All About Aging**   27

Fact: Often sold by dermatologists and other physicians, but sometimes available from retail stores and other sources, some of these products may contain stabilized and higher concentrations of various ingredients. Some doctors will make these products available to their patients out of convenience, while others may be selling them because of the profit incentive. Whether or not these creams, lotions, and serums will have any extra benefits for your skin will depend on the actual ingredients and their levels of concentration.

MOST COMMONLY ASKED QUESTIONS

Question: What is the best "anti-aging" cream I can use?

Answer: The best cream you can use during the day is one that contains a sunscreen with an SPF of 15 or higher to prevent further sun damage. If you are looking for a cream that has other ingredients in it, you could select one that has vitamin C (listed as active and stable) in it for the daytime (wearing it under your sunscreen), and in the evening you could alternate between using a mild alpha hydroxy acid and a cream that contains vitamin A.

Question: If a cream is expensive, does it mean it's better than a lower-priced one?

Answer: No. Most of the larger cosmetic companies incorporate the costs of packaging, retail space, and advertising of their products into the price. These expenses are all reflected in the tremendously marked-up price that you are paying at cosmetic counters. Those glossy, full-page ads you see in magazines don't come cheap, and it is you—the consumer—who is ultimately paying for them.

Question: My doctor sells cosmetics at his/her office. Are they better than other products?

Answer: There is no guarantee that the cosmetic products you are purchasing from your physician are any better than those sold at cosmetic counters, spas, on the television, or in drug or grocery stores. While there are some physician-marketed products that are unique and worthwhile in their formulations, you must remember that doctors are making money selling these products. It is up to you to analyze the ingredients and their concentration in order to make an informed decision as to whether the products would be of any benefit to your particular needs.

Question: I've tried so many different types of acne products over the years and nothing seems to help. Is there anything I can use to improve it?

Answer: Acne is essentially hormonal and genetic in nature. Although it usually occurs at the time of puberty, it can also flare up in adulthood, and is especially common when there are hormonal changes in the body, such as pregnancy or going on and off the birth control pill. Anti-acne creams can sometimes help, but your treatment should begin with a visit to a dermatologist, who will most likely prescribe antibiotics, the birth control pill, an oral medication such as Accutane, or other types of treatments, including Blu-U with Levulan and Smoothbeam laser (see Chapter 3, "Nonablative Resurfacing of the Skin").

Chapter 3

Nonablative
Resurfacing of the Skin

To understand the aging process and what treatments are best for us individually, we must first understand the basic components of skin, which is made up of three main layers. The outermost and hardest layer is called the stratum corneum, which is primarily comprised of dead skin cells. Underneath the stratum corneum is the epidermis, and beneath the epidermis is the dermis. Below it all is a cushioning layer of fat, which pads our faces (and bodies), giving them added protection.

The skin is actually the body's largest organ and is designed to keep anything harmful, such as environmental toxins, bacteria, and ultraviolet rays, away from our other life-maintaining organs. Miraculous in its composition, the skin is also made up to keep important vital fluids such as blood and water in the body. Because of this secure makeup, it is very difficult, if not impossible, for most over-the-counter cosmetics to actually penetrate the skin.

Being the outermost layers, the stratum corneum and underlying epidermis protect the body, and it is here that we first notice sun damage in the form of roughness. The sun will also eventually bring on pigmentation changes such as brown spots by causing abnormalities of the epidermis, where some of our pigment-producing cells reside. It is interesting to note that the entire lifespan of the epidermis is short-lived, with new cells replacing the dead cells on the surface approximately every three weeks.

As important as the stratum corneum and the epidermis are, it is in the dermis where the most significant aging process takes place. Made up of a fluid base known as hyaluronic acids, an elastic protein called elastin, and a fibrous protein named collagen, the dermis is by far the most significant structural element of our skin. It is here where nerves, hair follicles, and sweat and oil glands reside. Yet, in determining the way our skin looks and feels to the touch, it is the elastin and collagen that play the biggest role.

Elastin gives the skin its tone and elasticity, while collagen, the building block of the skin, provides it with strength. Working together in a woven fashion throughout the dermis, both the elastin and collagen have the ability to constantly regenerate themselves, but as we age and expose ourselves to pollutants, ultraviolet rays, and other harmful toxins, these vital elements of the skin gradually weaken, break down, and are eventually depleted. The degeneration of collagen causes the skin to wrinkle and also allows blood vessels to dilate, causing broken blood vessels to appear on the skin. Aside from the formation of lines, other outward signs of the loss of collagen and elastin are yellowing, sagging, thin, loose skin with deep furrows, and the inability to heal itself of wounds as quickly as it once did.

Fortunately, there are a number of nonablative (meaning nonsurgical) or noninjurious ways to correct these outward signs of aging and damage to the overall skin on the face. Involving little or no downtime, these noninvasive techniques lightly resurface the skin, giving varying results depending on the procedure. Most are done in a dermatologist's office, and

can be performed in well under an hour with little or no side effects. As we age four main events occur:
1. Sun damage in the form of brown spots, broken blood vessels, yellowing of the skin, larger pores, wrinkles, and changes in texture.
2. Wrinkles caused by movement and non movement.
3. Folds which appear along the nose, mouth, and between the brows.
4. Sagging with jowls and drooping of the brow.

Skin Rejuvenation Options

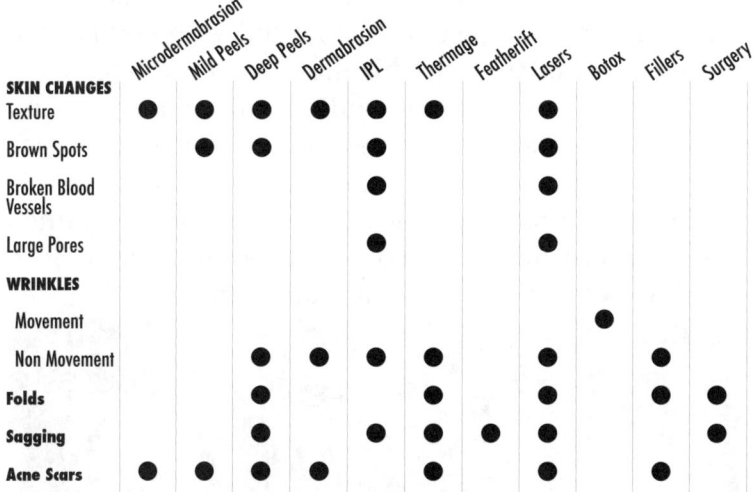

SKIN CHANGES	Microdermabrasion	Mild Peels	Deep Peels	Dermabrasion	IPL	Thermage	Featherlift	Lasers	Botox	Fillers	Surgery
Texture	●	●	●	●	●	●		●			
Brown Spots		●	●		●			●			
Broken Blood Vessels					●			●			
Large Pores					●			●			
WRINKLES											
Movement									●		
Non Movement		●	●	●	●			●		●	
Folds			●			●		●		●	●
Sagging			●		●	●	●	●			●
Acne Scars	●	●	●	●		●		●			

MICRODERMABRASION

Background: Microdermabrasion, which minimally reduces fine lines and helps to treat age spots, acne, and other surface imperfections, is a gentle way to exfoliate the top layer of the skin. First used by the ancient Egyptians, who incorporated rocks, sand, and other abrasive natural materials to take off the outer layer of skin cells, the technique has remained relatively unchanged for thousands of years. Recently, however, a hygienic method of spraying the face with fine crystals, and then vacuuming off the residue was developed in Italy.

Some cosmetic companies still sell products that contain jagged pieces of pumice, ground nuts, and other raw materials to exfoliate the skin. While, in fact, abrasive substances will remove the outer layer of dead skin cells to reveal newer skin cells underneath, using these types of harsh products can actually harm the skin by causing microscopic tears and lacerations.

Technique: Microdermabrasion, as opposed to dermabrasion, which is a surgical procedure involving the use of a rotary instrument to plane the skin, is done superficially and will not penetrate through the epidermis, therefore leaving no open sores or oozing. Performed without an anaesthetic, either in an esthetic spa or a doctor's office, the skin is first cleansed, and then sprayed with fine crystals. Although some technicians use natural salts, sodium carbonate, calcium, organic crystals, or other minerals, aluminum salt is considered to be superior. After the skin surface has been lightly abraded, the crystals and dead skin cells are then vacuumed off, using an instrument with sterile, disposable nozzles. The procedure takes about half an hour to complete.

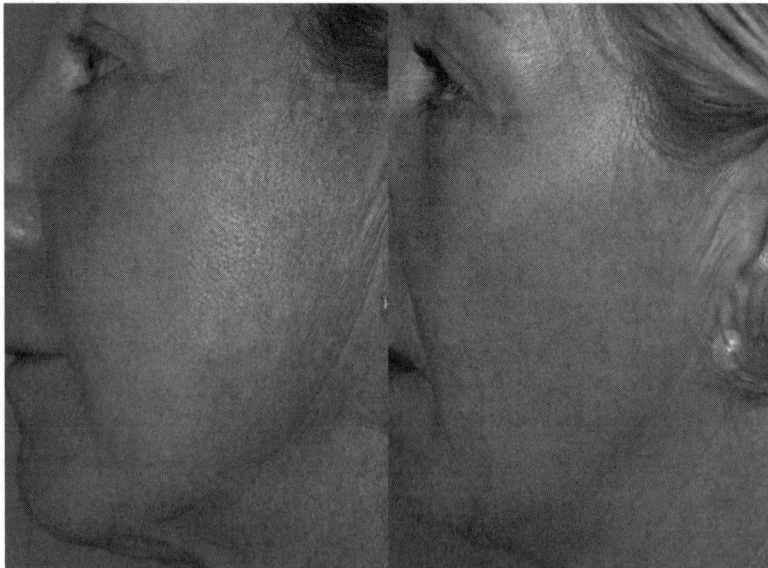

Smoother skin by microdermabrasion.

Chapter 3| Nonablative Resurfacing of the Skin 33

Downtime: There is little or no downtime involved in the procedure and most patients will return to work or their regular routine immediately afterwards.

Complications: After microdermabrasion, the skin may be somewhat red and swollen, but this will dissipate within 12 hours. Other than a rare allergic reaction to the crystals, you should expect little or no complications. If you have a tendency towards cold sores, the procedure may stimulate the herpes simplex virus, causing an outbreak. In order to avoid this, an antiviral medication, prescribed by your doctor, should be taken before the treatment.

Post-treatment: Wear a sunscreen with an SPF of 15 for several days afterwards.

Results: Although there are claims that microdermabrasion will remove wrinkles, acne scars, stretch marks, correct pigmentation changes, and decrease pore size, these type of dramatic results are unfounded. The truth is that the procedure will make your skin glow and give it a finer and smoother look and feel. Because of the mechanical effects of microdermabrasion, which exfoliate the stratum corneum, the process also stimulates collagen production and increases the amount of collagen deposition into the skin. When performed on a regular basis, the technique also thickens the epidermis over time. An extremely gentle procedure, microdermabrasion may also be done on the neck, chest, arms, and hands with few complications.

Ideal Candidate: If you do not have deep wrinkles or much sun damage, but do have dull-looking skin, microdermabrasion will address this. If you are older and have more damaged skin and wrinkles, microdermabrasion will provide subtle changes, lessening the appearance of fine lines, lightening some pigmentation, and giving a rosy glow to your skin. Acne scars will be reduced only slightly. Microdermabrasion is a great "pick-me-up" for dull and tired-looking skin.

How Often: Microdermabrasion should be performed every six weeks for six times, and then every three to four months

afterwards. A single treatment is insufficient and there will be few noticeable changes to the skin.
Cost: $100 to $200 per session.

SUPERFICIAL CHEMICAL PEELS

Background: Giving many of the same results as microdermabrasion, where the top layer of the stratum corneum is removed, superficial chemical peels were probably first used by Egyptian and Roman women. Utilizing acids found in foods that had fermented or soured, such as fruits and milk, they would apply the substances in an attempt to slough off the outermost layer of the skin. However, because the acid content of a natural peel wouldn't be strong enough to remove all of the dead skin cells, only a mild form of exfoliation would take place. In the early 1900s, it is recorded that chemical peels using a "secret formulation" were performed on American and European women at spas, and the various type of peels developed from that era onward. In the 1950s an extremely deep method called the phenol peel was invented. Currently, there are various strengths of chemical peels available, and the medium and deeper types of peels will be discussed in Chapter 4, "Medium and Deep Chemical Peels and Dermabrasion." It should be noted that certain cosmetic companies claim to have products that peel the skin, but without the higher concentration of alpha hydroxy acids in their formulations, these cosmetics simply exfoliate some of the dead skin cells and the resulting glow to the skin will only last a few hours.

Currently there are four types of superficial peels on the market. The mildest uses a concentration of a 30 to 50 percent alpha hydroxy or glycolic acid and gives an extremely superficial peel. For a slightly deeper peel, beta hydroxy or salicylic acids are used, while a Jessner's peel combines all of these acids, and penetrates a little deeper. To improve hyperpigmentation or brown spots on the skin, a Kojic acid peel is available.

Chapter 3| Nonablative Resurfacing of the Skin

Technique: Performed in a doctor's office or in an esthetic spa, the skin is first thoroughly cleansed to remove any oils. Your hair will be tied back and covered, and your eyes will be protected with pads. It is also recommended that you keep your eyes closed during any type of peel, no matter how mild. Utilizing one or more of the above types of acids, the liquid chemical is applied to the skin for as little as one to two minutes or for as long as ten minutes, depending on the amount of peeling desired.

Downtime: Since only the outermost layers of the skin are treated, there is little or no downtime, although depending on the strength of the peel, your face may be a little redder than normal for some time after treatment.

Complications: Superficial chemical peels are usually safe for anyone with light skin, although minimal redness may occur for a few days afterwards. Anyone with a darker complexion may get significant pigmentation changes, such as pale or dark patches, after the peel. The main complication of this treatment (as in microdermabrasion) may be an activation of herpes simplex on the face if the patient has a tendency towards cold sores. An antiviral medication should be taken prior to the procedure in order to prevent stimulation of the virus. A lesser complication would be patchy healing caused by pigmentation abnormalities. With a Jessner's peel, your skin may become very dry and small cracks may appear. An emollient moisturizer or Vaseline can be applied to counteract the dryness.

Post-treatment: It is recommended that you wear a sunscreen with an SPF of 25 or greater for several days after treatment because your skin will be more sensitive than usual to heat and light. Especially after being treated with a Jessner's peel, you should not apply any topical medications that you may have been using prior to your peel, such as Retin-A, Renova, or gylcolic acid.

Results: Claims that a superficial chemical peel will remove wrinkles and acne scars and reduce the size of the pores is untrue. Although some lightening of abnormal pigmentation

may occur, especially with the Kojic peel, the main noticeable improvement will be in the texture of the skin, which will be smoother looking and glowing.
Ideal Candidate: This procedure is suitable for a younger person with minimal sun damage and wrinkles. A superficial chemical peel is not for someone who wants to remove wrinkles or acne scars, or those persons with a darker complexion, because of the associated complications.
How Often: To gain noticeable results, a superficial chemical peel should be repeated every six weeks for three times, and then every three to four months thereafter. A Kojic acid peel should be repeated every four weeks until the brown spots begin to lighten and the skin tone evens out.
Cost: $100 to $200 per treatment.

PHOTO FACIALS (IPL) WITH OR WITHOUT LEVULAN

Background: Intense pulse light—photo facials—recently came on the market because of the development of a broad band pulse light source. Used to treat the entire face, neck and chest area, the intense pulse light is different from the traditional laser in that it operates in a spectrum of light, while the laser uses light in one wavelength. Containing all the wavelengths of the laser (i.e., wavelengths that target either brown, red, water, or collagen), the intense pulse band of light performs on a nanometre scale of 500 to 1200, and your doctor will discern where in the band you need to be treated.

Intense pulse light therapy is often used in conjunction with a pretreatment medication called Levulan. Approved by the FDA and Health and Welfare Canada for the treatment of sun-damaged skin, Levulan contains a 20 percent solution of aminolevulinic acid (ALA). Found naturally in the body, ALA is actually a precursor for hemoglobin synthesis, meaning that without it, we would be unable to produce red blood cells to carry oxygen. When used with photo rejuvenation,

Chapter 3| **Nonablative Resurfacing of the Skin** 37

Levulan will boost the light therapy and enhance the results. In fact, treatment without the use of the medication will usually require five sessions as opposed to three if the medication is used.

There is another form of IPL called Fotofacial RF™ (ELOS - combined energy technology using bi-polar radio frequency and light), which combines intense pulse light with radio frequency and claims to provide superior results.

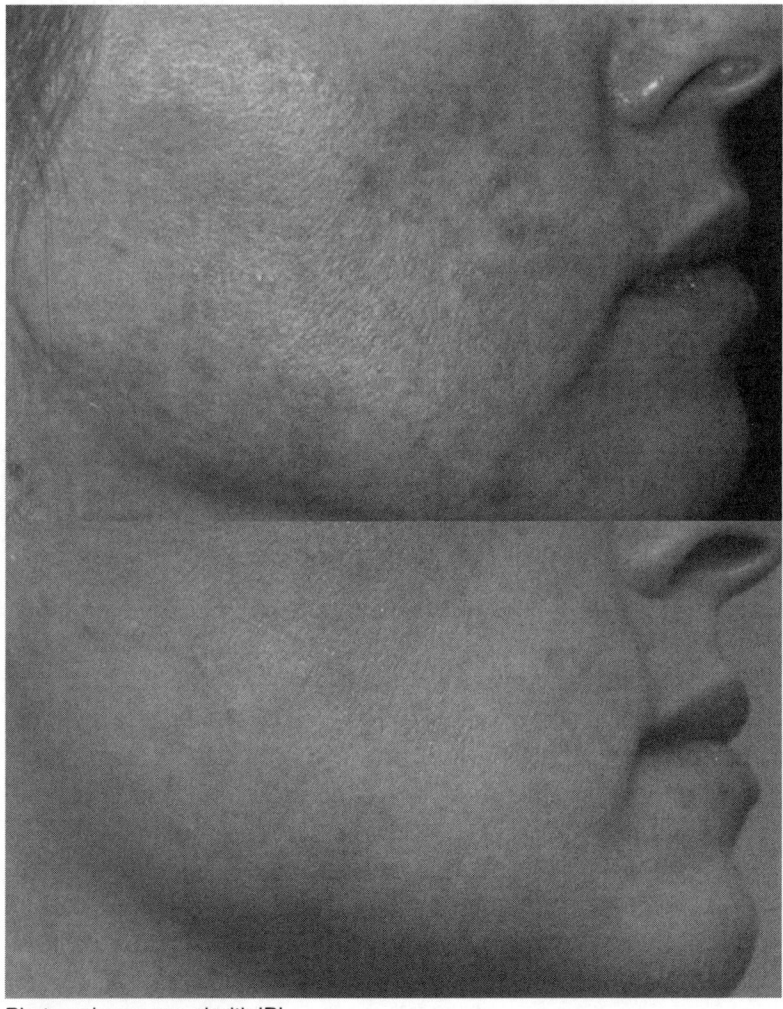

Photo-aging reversed with IPL.

Technique: If done in conjunction with Levulan, the doctor will prescribe a pretreatment of the medication prior to your IPL session. Either natural or artificial tanning should be avoided before the procedure, and in fact, most doctors will not treat recently tanned skin. Taking about an hour to perform on a cleansed face wearing no makeup, and usually using no anaesthesia other than a cooling tip on the instrument, a photo facial should only be performed by a doctor or a trained nurse under the supervision of a doctor. Your face will be coated with a gel-like substance and you will be given protective eye gear to wear. As the instrument transmits a series of light rays, you will see bright flashes as the intense pulse light hits the skin, and there may be a slight stinging sensation.

Downtime: Approximately twenty-four hours. Most patients return to work the next day. If Levulan is used, up to one week.

Complications: You may be a little red and swollen after treatment. Any brown spots that you had prior to the procedure may crust right off the skin. Some patients continue to swell and crust the next day, but any of these side effects usually clear up within twenty-four hours. If you have a tendency towards cold sores, the treatment may stimulate the herpes simplex virus, and an antiviral medication should be taken prior to the procedure.

Post-treatment: Wear a sunscreen containing an SPF of 30 or higher for several days afterwards.

Results: Claims are that photo facials will decrease broken blood vessels and pigmentation by 70 percent, and reduce the size of wrinkles and pores by 50 percent. While it dramatically improves the colour damage in your skin by decreasing freckles, evening out mottled pigmentation, and erasing broken blood vessels, it will only improve wrinkles and pores slightly. There will also be a moderate tightening effect on the overall skin. The result of a photo facial is most dramatic, especially after a couple of treatments, and offers a vast improvement over other nonablative treatments previously offered by a dermatologist. Your sun-damaged skin will take on a "peaches and cream" look, mimicking that of the skin under the breasts. Another

Chapter 3| **Nonablative Resurfacing of the Skin** 39

advantage to a photo facial is that it will make the epidermis thicker by stimulating collagen formation.

Ideal Candidate: The person who would most benefit from intense pulse light therapy is someone with light skin colour with significant sun damage on the skin, manifested by increased pigmentation such as freckles, sun spots and broken blood vessels.

How Often: Once every four weeks for a total of five sessions (without Levulan) or three sessions (with Levulan). Thereafter, once a year to maintain results.

Cost: $500 to $700 per session (without Levulan), $1,000 per session (with Levulan).

BLU-U THERAPY

Background: Used to treat acne and sun damaged skin, and best used in conjunction with Levulan medication, Blu-U is a type of light therapy, that should be performed by a doctor. By applying Levulan and then directing the Blu-U, which is set at a certain wavelength and will emit a blue light, the process will activate the Levulan and destroy acne bacteria. It also decreases the size of the sebaceous glands, and has the ability to remove some precancerous growths.

Technique: Approximately thirty minutes to an hour prior to the Blu-U session, Levulan will be applied to your cleansed, makeup-free face. Taking about eight minutes to perform, the Blu-U will then be directed to the treatment area. Expect some discomfort during the procedure because of the nature of the Levulan solution, which will usually improve immediately after treatment.

Downtime: Two to seven days.

Complications: During and after the procedure, there may be some discomfort that can last for up to twenty-four hours. There may also be some redness and swelling of the acne and the surrounding skin. While the swelling will usually subside within two to seven days, the reddening may take up to a month to disappear. The skin will also be extremely sensitive

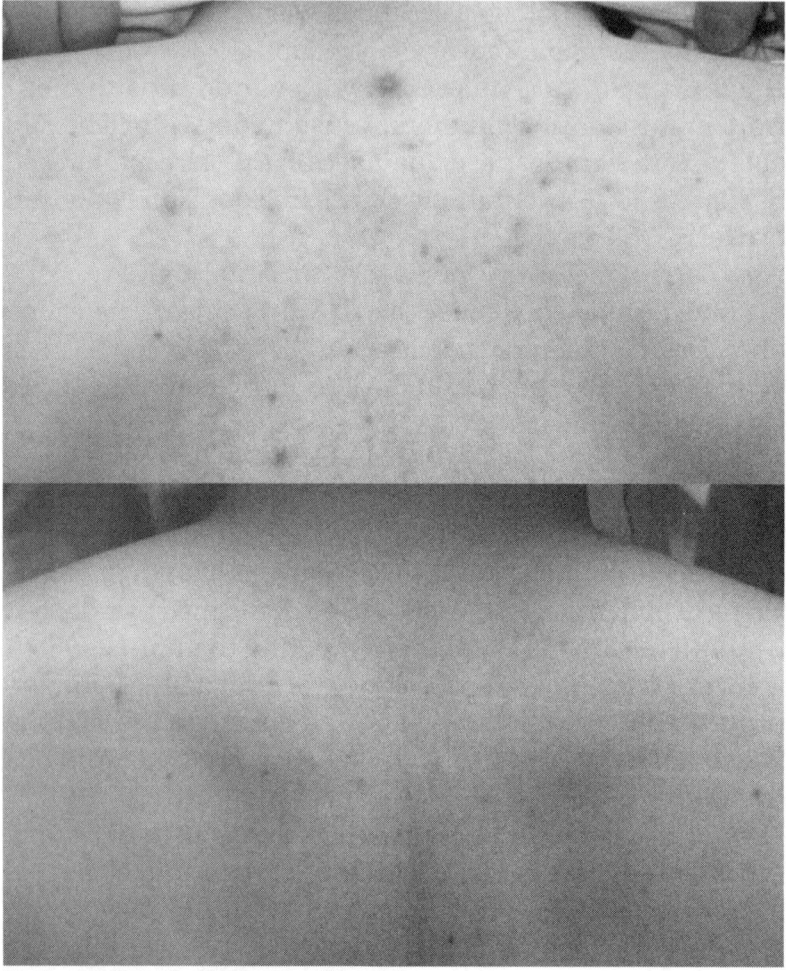

Back acne cleared with Blu-U and Levulan.

to sunlight after this procedure, for a day or so. Any precancerous growths will crust before falling off.

Post-treatment: In order to avoid any sunlight, it is recommended that you stay indoors for a period of twenty-four hours after the procedure. Thereafter, you must wear a sunscreen with an SPF of 45 or higher for several weeks.

Results: With multiple treatments, Blu-U therapy with Levulan will improve acne, remove pre-cancerous growths, and, although not as effective as intense pulse light photo facials,

will improve red and brown spots caused by sun damage.
Ideal Candidate: If you have precancerous growths or any form of acne, including comedonal (blackheads and whiteheads), papular, pustular or cystic, this procedure will be of benefit to you.
How Often: To clear adult acne, you will require up to four treatments every six weeks. Adolescents may require further treatment in six months to a year. To remove precancerous growths, you will require one to three sessions.
Cost: $500 per session.

NONABLATIVE LASERS

Background: Different from the traditional laser, (see Chapter 5, "Laser Techniques"), a nonablative laser does not cause injury to the skin. Used over the past decade, there are several types of lasers that fall into this category, but the most popular are the N-Lite System, which operates on a wavelength of 595 nanometres, the CoolTouch, which uses a 1,320 nanometre wavelength and the Smoothbeam, which operates on the highest wavelength of 1,450 nanometres. All of these lasers are mildly effective in treating fine lines and wrinkles around the eyes and mouth, and are also used for removing superficial acne scars. These lasers work to lightly resurface the skin by minimally heating up the epidermis and dermis. As the laser light passes through the skin, and the water absorbs the heat, any collagen in the area is also heated, causing it to remodel or reshape and get somewhat tighter. While not as effective as the ablative type lasers, noninjurious laser treatment is growing increasingly popular because it does provide positive results with little or no recovery time.

It should be noted that a red laser light is currently being sold to consumers called a soft laser light energy skin treatment. The manufacturer claims that it will wake up skin cells to produce new collagen, make skin glow, and treat acne, psoriasis, burns, scars, bruising, wrinkles, and spider veins. It also claims that there is no heat involved and no typical laser "zapping." Since all lasers work by heating up the skin, it is our opinion that this device would seem to be of little or no benefit.

Technique: About a half hour before the procedure, the doctor (or nurse) may apply a topical local anaesthetic such as EMLA to the face. This is a precaution to safeguard against the stinging sensation that occurs when the laser is fired. If you are sensitive and your doctor has not recommended the anaesthetic, you may want to suggest having it applied. Once the procedure is underway, you will feel a sting much like the sensation of having a rubber band snapped against the skin. You will be wearing protective eyewear, and the actual laser treatment will take about half an hour.

Downtime: Approximately twelve hours, but you should be able to return to work the next day.

Complications: You will probably be a little red after the procedure, and there may be some pigment change for a few days, but any discoloration will fade away over time.

Post-treatment: Because your skin may be sensitive after the procedure, sun exposure and abrasive skin care products should be avoided for four to six weeks after treatment. A sunscreen containing an SPF of 25 should be worn for several weeks afterwards.

Results: Nonablative laser resurfacing will have a mild effect on fine wrinkles, especially around the lower eyelid area and around the mouth, and will also diminish the size of acne scars. Since this type of laser resurfacing stimulates collagen production, the epidermis of the skin will thicken somewhat. The procedure will also even out the texture and colour of rough skin, and can improve superficial acne scars. If the Smoothbeam laser is used, the pore size will decrease because unlike the other types of nonablative lasers, the Smoothbeam actually diminishes the size of the oil glands.

Ideal Candidate: If you have fine wrinkles, especially under the eyes and around the mouth, rough skin that is losing texture and colour, and your pore size is becoming larger,

you will benefit from the various types of nonablative laser resurfacing. Those with superficial acne scars will also see some diminishment.
How Often: Although up to six treatments may be required, there will be a noticeable improvement after the first treatment. Thereafter, any visual betterment will be gradual.
Cost: $300 to $500 per treatment.

FRAXEL

Background: Because this is a new system, we have no clinical experience using the Fraxel and the following information is based on the manufacturer's claims.

Offering many of the positive effects of ablative laser resurfacing (see Chapter 5, "Laser Techniques"), without the complications and downtime, Fractional Photothermolysis (Fraxel) is a laser system that produces microscopic thermal wounds to the skin that are separated by areas of unaffected tissue. These untreated areas contain viable cells that will rapidly renew the outer skin layers to achieve photo rejuvenation, while the tiny micro-thermal wounds penetrate into the dermis to remodel the collagen.

Technique: A blue tinted substance will first be applied to your cleansed skin, followed by a topical anaesthetic, which will take approximately forty-five minutes to become fully effective. The actual session involves a robotic-type hand piece that glides across the skin as if it were painting it. The blue tint darkens the tiny folds of the skin, allowing the robotic device to read the contours of the area and perform precise treatment. Expect some discomfort during the procedure, which will feel like a prickling sensation.

Downtime: Little or none.

Complications: There will be some mild swelling that will subside within twenty-four hours, and redness that may take a few days to disappear. There is a very low risk of infection and/or scarring.

Post-treatment: None.

Results: With multiple treatments, there will be increased collagen production and a gradual remodelling of the skin, which will appear firmer and tighter within a one to three month period.

Ideal Candidate: If you have skin that has been damaged from the sun and has some drooping, especially around the jowls, you may benefit from this procedure.

How Often: Four to six sessions, spaced from five to seven days apart.

Cost: Because this procedure has only recently been introduced, costs are still to be determined.

THERMAGE

Background: Also known as ThermaLift, Radiothermoplasty, and ThermaCool, thermal plastic contouring works with radio frequency energy to heat up the collagen in the dermis, while cooling and protecting the epidermis. This causes the underlying structure in your skin to immediately contract or tighten, and the collagen to regenerate over time.

Technique: You will most likely be given a mild analgesic painkiller and sedative upon arriving at the doctor's office. As an extra precaution, an anaesthetic cream may be topically applied over the cleansed face. The procedure takes over an hour to do the full facial area. Using a small instrument equipped with a cooling tip that sprays the skin before, during, and after each pulse of radio frequency, the doctor, (or trained nurse under the supervision of a doctor), will touch the tip of the device over all areas of your face. As the radio frequency energy is converted into electricity and passes into your skin, it will generate heat with the resistance of the skin. At this point, you will experience an intense warming sensation that will sting, but it will be immediately followed by a cooling sensation. It is this generation of heat which causes the collagen to remodel.

Chapter 3| **Nonablative Resurfacing of the Skin** 45

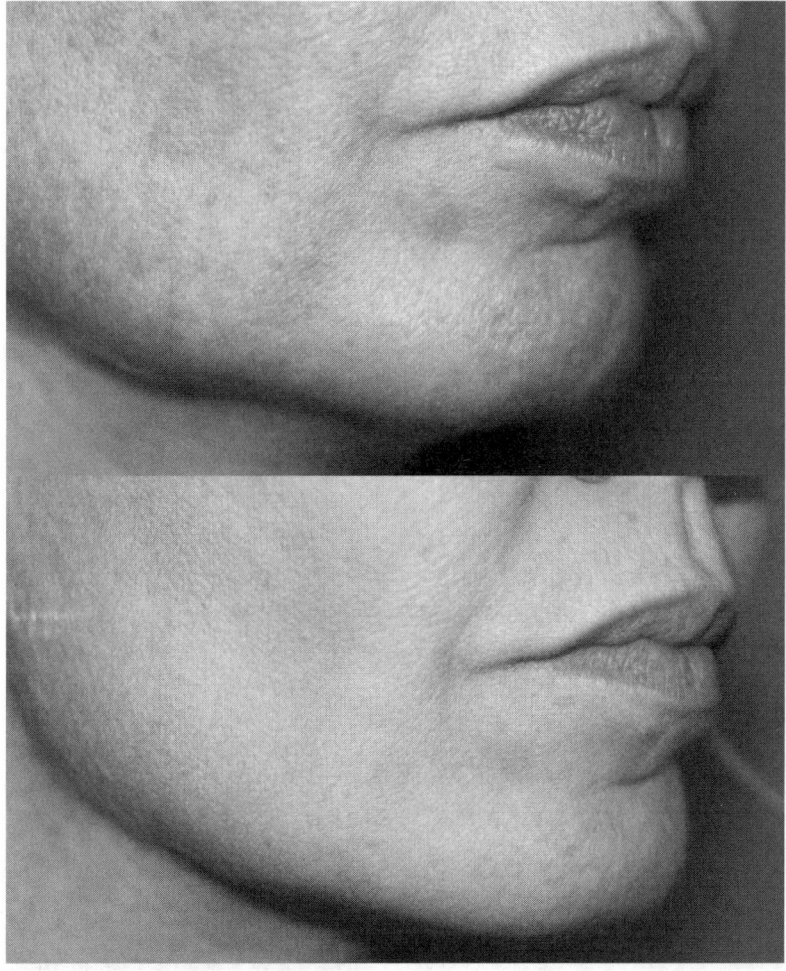

Jawline enhancement with Thermage.

Downtime: Most people return to their regular routine immediately following the procedure.

Complications: There may be some redness similar to a mild sunburn immediately following treatment. There is also a possibility of swelling. Although unlikely, some patients experience a waffling of the skin while healing, where some areas have tightened more than others, but this can usually be corrected with massage.

Post-treatment: None.

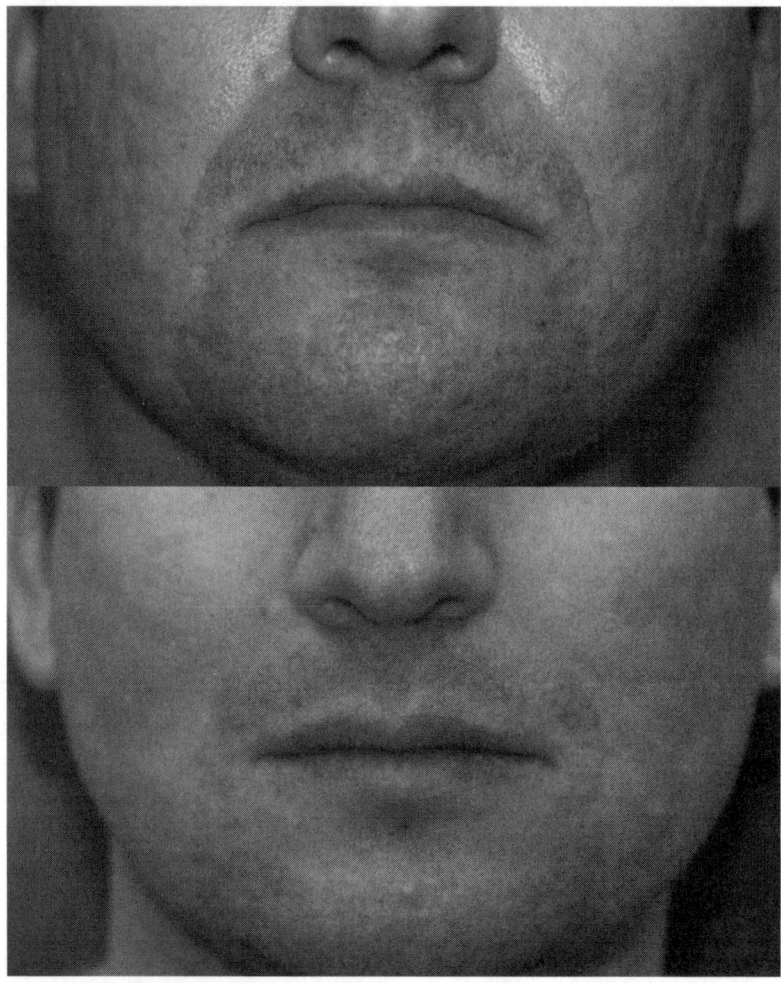

Acne scar improvement with Thermage.

Results: Although the underlying structure of the skin is immediately tightened upon application of the radio frequency energy, visual results will not be seen for a couple of months. Gradually, your skin will appear smoother and tighter, with the tightening process removing any fine wrinkles. This procedure works especially well on wrinkles around the eyes (called the periorbital area). After a few more months, you will also begin to notice a lift to the skin. Overall, this procedure has the capacity to remove five years from your face.

Chapter 3| **Nonablative Resurfacing of the Skin** 47

Ideal Candidate: If you are considering a surgical facelift because you are noticing drooping, especially in the jowl or brow area, have deep marionette lines (the ones that run from the corner of the mouth to the chin) and also have fine lines and wrinkles, this procedure will provide excellent results. As it tightens the skin, it will also improve some forms of acne scarring. You must remember, however, that these results will not be noticeable right away. Also note that this procedure will not change the colour or pigmentation of your skin like a photo facial would.

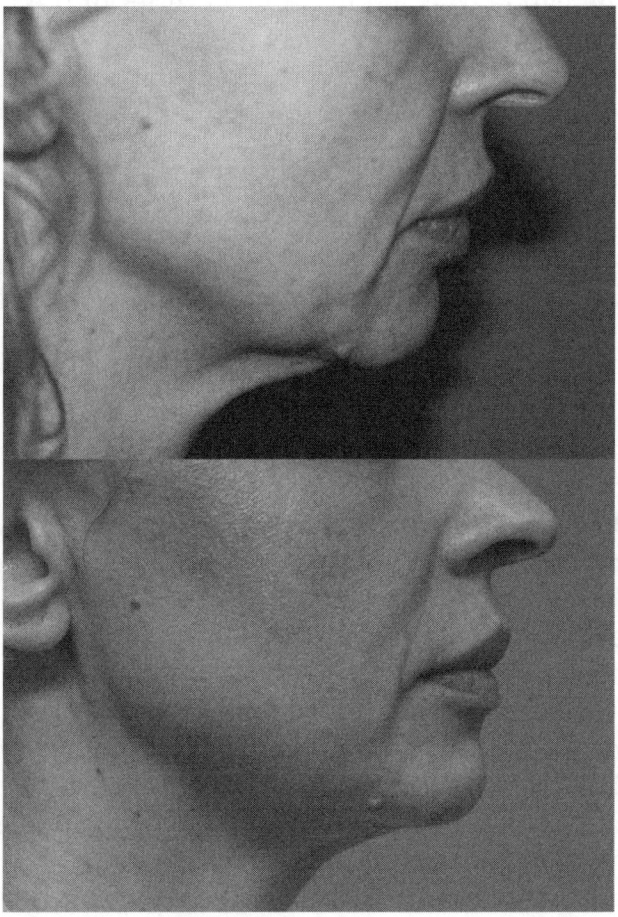

Jowl correction with Thermage.

How Often: Thermage need only be performed once on the average patient in order to obtain significant results. However, those with more looseness in their faces may require two treatments before any results will be noticeable.
Cost: $1,700 to $2,000 for the lower or upper half of the face. $2,800 to $3,500 for the entire face.

PAN G™ LIFT

We have no clinical experience using Pan G ™ and the following information is based on the manufacturer's claims.

The Pan G ™ is a non-surgical series of treatments which claim to produce a "facelift like" effect by applying radio frequency energy, high voltage galvanic electrical currents and high frequency ultra sound. The patient must commit to twenty treatments over a ten week period, then to a maintenance program which will require a visit to the doctor every four to six weeks.

The system has not been accepted by most plastic surgeons or cosmetic dermatologists and is available only in a few centres in North America.

FEATHERLIFT

Background: The Featherlift technique was developed by a Moscow-based surgeon by the name of Marlen Sulamanidze in 1999. Introduced to the North American market in 2003, the procedure involves inserting a series of hollow needles into the face and then threading a feathered suture through the needle and tightening it, which has a lifting affect. This technique is an excellent alternative to a face and brow lift for those who are beginning to experience a looseness of skin on the face and neck. Although there isn't the pain or downtime associated with traditional surgery, there also isn't the same dramatic results. Instead, Featherlift provides more subtle benefits that are seen over a period of time.
Technique: The doctor will first mark the face where the needles are to be inserted. A local anaesthetic is used. After the needles

are put in place in either a zigzag or arched pattern, 5 to 18 centimetres of intradermal suspension thread is inserted into the needle, which is then removed. As the thread is tightened, the underlying tissue of the skin will lift. Tiny feathers or barbs that run along the thread help to hold up the lifted area by attaching themselves to subcutaneous fat. Once the Featherlift procedure has been completed, surgical tape is applied over the area. The entire treatment, including the application of anaesthetic, should take no longer than one hour. Upon leaving the doctor's office, you will be given an ice pack to counteract the swelling.

Downtime: Three to five days.

Complications: There will be some mild swelling and discomfort during the first couple of days, and you will most likely notice a prickly sensation, which will also subside within a few days. Although bruising can last for up to two weeks, it can be easily covered with makeup. Other complications are rare, but can include puckering of the skin, which is corrected by gentle massage, or a thread working its way out of the entrance point, which the doctor can remedy by trimming and removing the thread.

Post-treatment: Ice packs should be applied to counteract any swelling, and a medication such as Tylenol can be taken to help with mild pain. The surgical tape can be removed three to five days after the procedure, but you should be careful not to apply any direct pressure to the area. It must be treated very gently for at least five days to allow the barbs to take hold. If you are considering other cosmetic procedures such as fillers, peels, or an eyelid lift, you must wait for at least six weeks.

Results: Some patients report seeing an immediate tightening of the skin, but in most cases results are more subtle and will be noticed after six weeks. Since collagen begins to form around the barbs after the operation, your skin will appear even firmer within a six-month period as collagen is regenerated.

Ideal Candidate: This procedure is best suited for those in the age range of thirty-five to fifty, who may be experiencing early sagging or drooping skin in the jowl, neck, or brow area.

How Often: The procedure need only be done once to achieve results, which can last for up to ten years. However, you may want to have the Featherlift performed in other areas that need attention.

Cost: $3,500 to $6,000 (depending on how much of an area is being done).

MOST COMMONLY ASKED QUESTIONS

Question: My esthetician promises me that microdermabrasion and glycolic acid peels will take away my wrinkles, decrease my pore size, improve my acne, and take away acne scarring. Is this true?

Answer: As a whole, microdermabrasion and mild glycolic acid peels are useful, but they will only improve the appearance of your skin slightly, giving it a glowing effect. They are very expensive, however, and must be repeated every few months in order to give any satisfying results.

Question: I used to be a sun worshipper, and even though I try to stay out of the sun now, I notice I have broken blood vessels and brown spots. What can I use to improve the appearance and texture of my skin?

Answer: The best treatment for this type of sun damage is intense pulse light photo facials, used in conjunction with Levulan, which will dramatically improve the effectiveness of the intense pulse light. After a period of time, you will see a significant improvement in the texture and colour of your skin.

Question: I am beginning to develop jowls, and I feel like I am looking old. How can I improve this?

Answer: Jowls, or the sagging of the skin along the jaw line, are basically a result of gravity. Thermage is very useful in slightly lifting the jowls, and the Featherlift technique will give a little more increase in lift, without undergoing major surgery. For any significant lift, however, you will have to consider a facelift.

Question: I have sun damaged skin that is wrinkling and sagging. What can I do?

Answer: The most effective treatment would be a combination of Thermage to improve the sagging of the skin, and intense pulse light to remove some of the signs of sun damage. Although the Fraxel laser treatment is new, and we have no clinical experience as of this writing, we are excited about its potential, as the manufacturer states the procedure will result in significant improvement in both the wrinkling and sagging of the skin with little downtime.

Question: My doctor has suggested that I have a photo facial with Levulan. Considering the extra cost, is the Levulan really necessary?

Answer: Yes. The results of an intense light photo facial are enhanced by performing the procedure in conjunction with the application of Levulan. Furthermore, the number of sessions will be significantly reduced.

Chapter 4

Medium and Deep

Chemical Peels and Dermabrasion

Even with the introduction of less invasive skin resurfacing procedures, certain ablative techniques that tend to harm the skin, such as medium to deep chemical peels and dermabrasion, still remain popular cosmetic treatments. People seem willing to risk the complications that can occur by abrading the skin deeply with manual devices and machines, in order to gain a more youthful looking complexion.

But you should be forewarned that these complications can be severe. There will be a risk of scarring, possible permanent lightening of the skin, and even associated health problems. Furthermore, the procedures can take weeks, and even months to heal. However, if done correctly by a qualified doctor, these invasive treatments can result in the removal of wrinkles, brown spots, and mild acne scarring. Obviously, methods that penetrate the skin less deeply will have lesser side effects and a shorter recovery period.

MEDIUM TO DEEP CHEMICAL PEELS
Trichloroacetic Acid (TCA) Peel

Background: Medium to deep chemical peels have been used by doctors since the 1950s. The most common of the medium-strength peels is known as the TCA. Unlike a superficial chemical peel that only removes the very outer layer of dead skin cells, this peel, which uses from 25 to 35 percent trichloroacetic acid, will take off the entire epidermis and part of the underlying dermis. To be performed only by a qualified physician, it is primarily used to improve pigmentation, wrinkles, and the texture and thickness of the skin. This procedure is not recommended for anyone with dark skin, as it could cause serious pigmentation changes.

Technique: For approximately five weeks prior to your procedure, your physician may prescribe a pre-op treatment of Retin-A or an alpha hydroxy acid, which will allow the chemical to absorb more readily into the skin. Upon arriving at the doctor's office, your face will be thoroughly cleansed and toned. Your hair will be tied back, and if you are wearing contact lenses, they will have to be removed. Vaseline will be applied around the lower eyes, on the lips, and around the nose to ensure the chemical stays away from those areas.

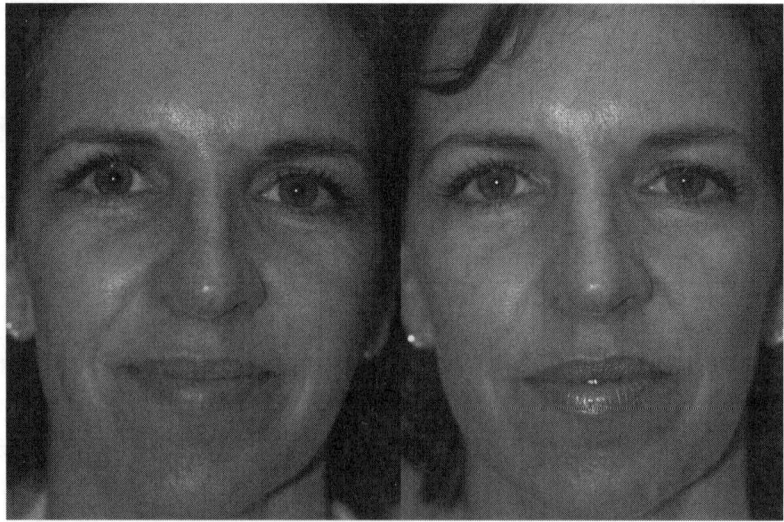

Skin rejuvenation with a mild TCA peel.

Protective eyewear must be worn, and you will be asked to keep your eyes closed during the procedure.

The procedure does not require anaesthesia. The chemical is usually applied in layers with cotton-tipped applicators, and will cause a white "frosting" to appear on the face within a couple of minutes. The skin will begin to feel warm and you will experience a burning sensation, which can be discomforting. Your doctor will most likely use a fan to cool the skin as the treatment continues. However, expect the stinging to last throughout the peel and diminish only after the procedure is completed. Your eyes may also tear up during treatment. Although unsettling, this is considered to be normal. After the procedure, which takes about fifteen minutes to complete, your face will be sprayed with thermal spring water to help calm the skin. Then a heavy moisturizer, along with a sunscreen with an SPF of 60, will be applied to your face.

Downtime: Five to ten days.

Complications: Immediately after the TCA peel, your skin will be swollen and very pink. Taking about a week to heal, the reaction can be from a mild peeling to a dramatic oozing, depending on the concentration of the TCA peel. The lesser the concentration, the lesser the reaction. The rosy tone of your skin will become very red, then slowly fade to dark brown. This is the stage when the skin begins to crust as it sheds itself of dead skin cells. It is also when you may become alarmed at the sight of your face. Within a very short time, however, new and much improved skin will be formed.

The main complication associated with this type of peel is the activation of the herpes simplex virus if you are prone to cold sores. If that is the case, you will be prescribed an antiviral medication prior to the procedure. A lesser risk would be pigmentation changes and chance of scarring.

Post-treatment: Cooling masks will be given to you when you leave the doctor's office, and should be applied as necessary. Wash your face using the mildest of cleansers, followed by Vaseline. As the skin heals, a heavy moisturizer and sunscreen containing an SPF of 60 should be used, although you must avoid direct sunlight and heat for at least two weeks after the peel. You may also apply Vaseline to any areas that are crusting and scabbing. You may resume your normal skincare regime ten days afterwards, although if you are using retinoids you should check first with your doctor.

Results: Removing any superficial acne blemishes, this procedure will also improve pigmentation, texture, and the thickness of the skin. Furthermore, surface wrinkles will be smoothed out.

Ideal Candidate: If you are in your thirties to fifties, have light skin that is sun damaged with fine wrinkles and some pigmentation, you would be a prime candidate for a TCA peel. Those with superficial acne scars will also benefit from the procedure.

How Often: After the first TCA peel, another one should be performed in six months, and then again in another six months.

Cost: $1,000–$2,000.

Phenol Peel

Background: Introduced in the early 1950s, a phenol peel is an extremely deep, invasive procedure that removes the epidermis and much of the dermis. With a reputation for having severe complications, this peel has the capacity to dramatically remove wrinkles and tighten the skin. Although older and more experienced physicians are still performing the phenol peel, you would be hard-pressed to find a younger doctor who would attempt one. Most modern physicians prefer laser resurfacing, which can provide the same positive benefits as a deep chemical peel, without the long recovery period and the higher risk of drastic side effects.

Because of the dangers involved with the phenol peel, it should only be performed by a qualified and very experienced doctor.

Technique: Prior to the procedure, the patient must undergo a series of pre-op testing of the heart, liver, and kidneys

Chapter 4 | Medium and Deep Chemical Peels and Dermabrasion

since the phenol chemical can be absorbed into the body, causing toxic internal damage. Furthermore, anyone with a history of heart disease should also be aware that the treatment can cause rapid heartbeat. Discuss your health history with your doctor before deciding on this peel.

To ensure that the peel will penetrate, your skin will be thoroughly cleansed and your hair will be tied back. Vaseline will then be applied around your eyes, nose, and mouth. Protective eyewear is worn over the eyes, which must be kept closed during the procedure. The chemical is applied evenly over the facial area, and you will experience a stinging sensation that will be at its worst as the frost develops over the skin. Some doctors will prescribe a mild sedative prior to the procedure to counteract the discomfort, while others may recommend taking two Aspirins an hour before the peel. Most physicians will use a fan to cool down the skin while the procedure is underway, which takes about an hour to complete.

Downtime: Pinkness may last six to eight weeks.

Complications: There can be significant side effects associated with a phenol peel. Because the entire top layer of the skin will fall off, your face will basically be a large open wound and will have to be treated as such. There will be extensive oozing and crusting, and the new skin will be very red for a prolonged period of time. Furthermore, the recovery time is very long and can take up to seven months before your skin has fully healed. There may also be scarring and a risk of infection. After you have recovered from this procedure, the skin will be almost alabaster in its tone because the melanin cells will have been destroyed in the process. The destruction of these cells will result in your inability to ever tan, or gain any colour back in the skin.

Post-treatment: Because the face will essentially be an open wound after the peel, there is an extensive post-op regime. Keep your head elevated for several days afterwards, and the wound must be routinely cleansed and dressed. Your doctor will prescribe exact treatment.

Results: Your skin will become very white afterwards and deep lines and wrinkles will have almost disappeared. There will also be a significant tightening to the skin comparable to a surgical facelift.
Ideal Candidate: If you have a fair complexion with extremely sun-damaged skin and severe wrinkles, you may be a candidate for this peel. Anyone with dark skin should not have a phenol peel.
How Often: Once.
Cost: $4,000.00.

DERMABRASION
Background: Based on the ancient theory that rough materials would remove the surface layer of the skin, revealing a rosier and younger looking complexion underneath, physicians first began to experiment with dermabrasion in the early 1900s. However, it wasn't until the 1950s that a machine was invented that used a rotating device to resurface the skin. As opposed to microdermabrasion (see Chapter 3, "Nonablative Resurfacing of the Skin"), which superficially exfoliates dead skin cells from the very outer surface, dermabrasion is a far more aggressive procedure that penetrates the second layer of skin. Often used on younger persons in an attempt to remove acne scars and older people with heavily photoaged skin, dermabrasion is considered to be a surgical procedure, and should only be performed by a qualified physician. While most modern doctors will perform microdermabrasion, many now prefer laser resurfacing to dermabrasion.
Technique: Because the skin is literally being sanded or planed with a rotating drill or wire brush, if the entire face is being treated, the procedure will be performed under a general anaesthetic. If a small, localized area is undergoing treatment to reduce acne scarring, for example, it may be done with a local anaesthetic. Cold in the form of bags or sprays will also be applied to the skin. Taking between ten and forty-five minutes, depending on the speed of your doctor

Chapter 4 | Medium and Deep Chemical Peels and Dermabrasion

and how deeply the skin is being abraded, the procedure will leave the skin red, raw, and oozing immediately afterwards. In most cases, an antibiotic ointment and dressing will be applied by the physician.

Downtime: One to six months. Older persons with thinning skin will take the longest time to heal.

Complications: If performed under a general anaesthetic, there will be the usual associated risks during the procedure. After the treatment, your face will be red, raw, oozing, and swollen. The redness will subside within a few days; however, your face will most likely remain swollen. Crusts will begin to form, and as the scabs begin to fall off, the treated area will be itchy. In some cases, scarring and infection can occur. Because the skin's top layer will have been removed, pigment cells may be destroyed in the process, which could leave the complexion very white and unable to tan afterwards. On the other hand, due to the excessive skin irritation, these same pigment cells may be stimulated, causing hyperpigmentation or a mottled look to the skin. During the procedure, the herpes simplex virus may also be stimulated, and an antiviral medication will be prescribed beforehand if you are susceptible to cold sores.

Post-treatment: Similar to after a phenol peel, your skin will have to be treated and dressed after a deep dermabrasion, and your doctor will prescribe your home care regime. Any exposure to sunlight must be avoided for at least six months, and thereafter a strong sunscreen must always be worn in order to decrease the risk of hyperpigmentation.

Results: Dermabrasion has the capacity to remove severe wrinkles and acne scars. It will also help to tighten the skin.

Ideal Candidate: Fair-skinned people with heavily sun-damaged, wrinkled, and loose skin, or diffuse acne scarring can benefit from dermabrasion. Dark-skinned people are not good candidates for this method of skin resurfacing.

How Often: Once.

Cost: $4,000

MOST COMMONLY ASKED QUESTIONS

Question: I have dark brown skin, and I was considering a medium-depth TCA peel, but I heard they may not be suitable for darker-skinned people. Is this true?

Answer: The darker the skin colour, the more careful you have to be with any procedure that causes deep peeling of the skin. Any such treatment will result in significant pigmentation changes, making the skin either whiter or darker after the peel.

Question: I have melasma, would a TCA peel help?

Answer: Melasma is an abnormal reaction of pigment cells to sun. It may be induced by hormonal changes, eg., the birth control pill or pregnancy. The mainstay of treatment is avoidance of sun and bleaching agents that contain hydroquinoine. A mild to moderate TCA peel may help in improving melasma.

Question: I have acne scarring. Would you recommend CO_2 laser resurfacing or dermabrasion?

Answer: Dermabrasion would be recommended for extremely severe acne scarring where deep pitting was evident. The dermabrasion may require repeat treatments and may be followed up with CO_2 laser and perhaps Thermage.

Question: I have dark skin. Would I benefit from a chemical peel?

Answer: A phenol or TCA peel would not be recommended due to the risk of hyperpigmentation for your skin, however, Kojic acid or Jessner's peels may be effective in improving fine lines and wrinkles and evening out your skin tone.

Chapter 5

Laser Techniques

The theory behind modern laser technology was first introduced by Einstein in 1917, but it wasn't until 1959, when a laser was invented that used a ruby crystal to produce red light, and that would go on to treat reddish coloured skin lesions. Best described by its acronym (light amplified stimulated emission of radiation), laser light is different from any other light form. While typical light is a spectrum of many wavelengths, laser light has only one wavelength, which can pass through the skin, heat it up, and destroy selective tissue.

Lasers require a substance such as carbon dioxide, erbium, a ruby, or alexandrite to generate the light, and are classified by this substance and the colour of light that is emitted from them. The argon gas laser, which produces a blue-green light, was once used to treat port wine stain birthmarks. Although they were somewhat successful at lightening the birthmark, the argon laser also caused severe scarring in the area being treated, and is not generally used in this day and age. It wasn't until the 1980s that selective photothermolysis, meaning light thermal (or heat) injury, was discovered. With this new form of laser technology, the targeted area would still absorb the light omitted from the laser, but only for a determined amount of time, resulting in the selected tissue being destroyed, leaving the surrounding skin intact.

There are three areas in the skin than can be targeted by laser light: hemoglobin or blood, melanin, and water. Pigment that has been introduced into the skin can also be targeted. Lasers that target hemoglobin can remove any red spots such as blood vessels and rosacea, while lasers that hit the melanin will treat brown spots and hair. When water is targeted, it will induce heat in the skin cells and work to repair wrinkles. Lasers will also target exogenous pigments such as tattoo pigments.

Because everything in the universe absorbs light at a different wavelength, where the laser is set in the band of light, or at how many nanometres, will determine what will be targeted in the skin. If the laser is set at 532 nanometers, it will just hit melanin, while hemoglobin will require a setting of 585 nanometres. 800 nanometres will strike melanin and destroy hair follicles, and if the laser is set at 1,064 nanometres, it targets both hemoglobin and melanin.

Due to the obvious complexity regarding the subject of lasers, and the severe and permanent damage that can occur if the procedure is not done correctly, it is extremely important that laser treatment be performed only by a qualified medical specialist.

Since various skin disorders and conditions can be treated by more than one type of laser, the following section will be classified by the problem, and then by the lasers that are most commonly used for treatment.

WRINKLES
Carbon Dioxide Laser

Background: Essentially vaporizing the top layer of the skin off the epidermis and applying heat directly into the dermis, which ultimately tightens up the collagen, the carbon dioxide laser (CO_2) has been used since the mid 1990s to remove wrinkles. Considered to give the most dramatic of results to photodamaged skin, the effects of this laser can also mimic a surgical facelift. However, because the CO_2 laser was being used by persons who were not properly trained or qualified, severe complications occurred. Subsequently, the popularity of the CO_2 laser has dropped as other less ablative techniques have been developed. It should be emphasized, however, that if used by a physician who is well trained in laser technology, the carbon dioxide laser will provide outstanding results. The two types of carbon dioxide lasers that are currently in use are the pulsed laser, with the brand name of UltraPulse, and the scan carbon dioxide laser, with the brand names FeatherTouch or SilkTouch.

Technique: The use of a CO_2 laser requires anaesthesia. If a small area is being treated, such as the wrinkles around the mouth or the eyes, a local anaesthetic will be sufficient, but if the entire face is being resurfaced, a general anaesthetic or a local with sedation administered intravenously is necessary, and the patient will essentially be asleep for the hour and a half that it will take for treatment. Even though this laser can be used directly under the eye to treat fine lines and wrinkles, protective eye shields must still be worn.

Downtime: You should be able to return to your normal routine in ten to twelve days. However, redness may last for up to six months to a year.

Complications: Because the treated area will be a large, open wound, it will ooze continuously for days, and unless properly cleansed there is a risk of infection. After it heals, the area will be very red for a prolonged period, but this will fade over time. There is also an increased risk of scarring using this laser. Furthermore, the area may heal lighter than normal and may never tan. Darker-skinned people may get even darker or lighter.

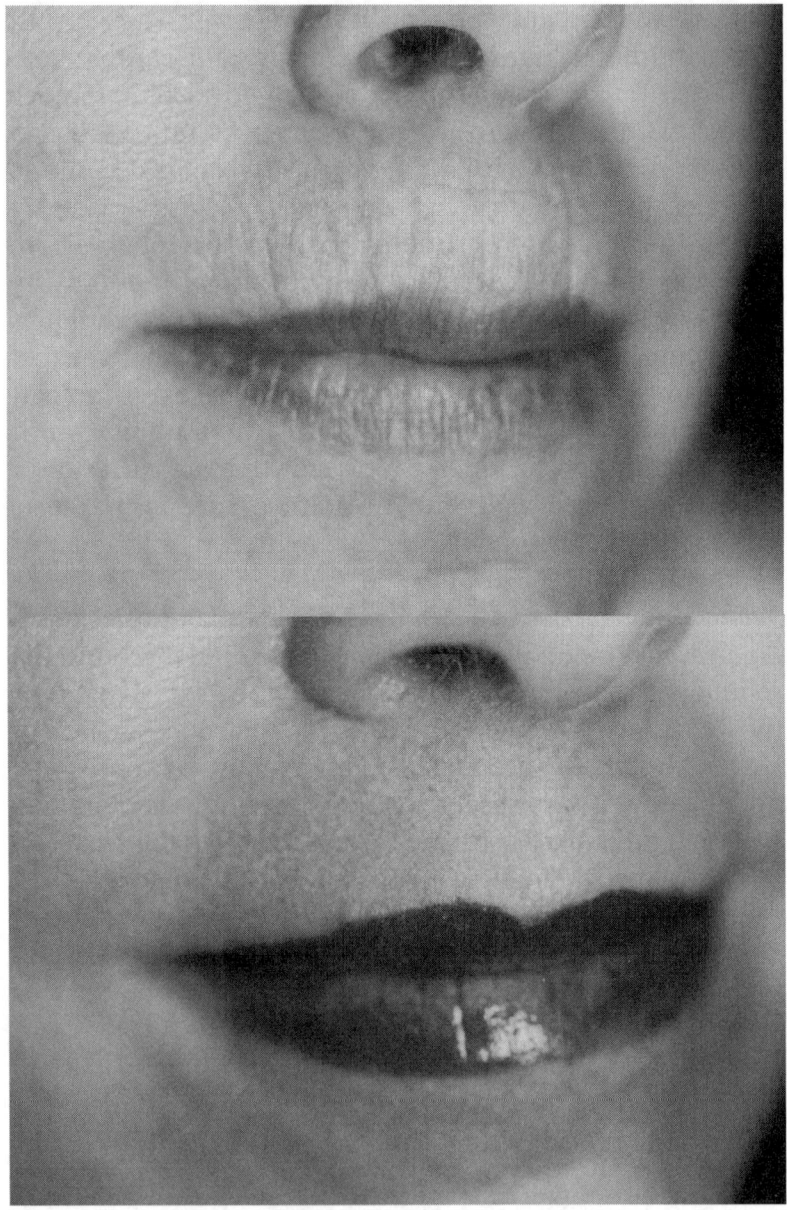

Laser wrinkle removal.

Chapter 5| **Laser Techniques** 65

Post-treatment: The area must be cleansed and dressed daily; your doctor will prescribe exact treatment. You must avoid sun exposure and wear a sunscreen with an SPF of 60 for at least six months after the procedure.

Results: There will be up to a 70 to 90 percent reduction in wrinkles and significant lifting and tightening of the skin.

Ideal Candidate: If you have severely photo-damaged skin with deep lines and sagging over the entire face, this is a technique worthy of consideration. It will also be of benefit to those who have wrinkles around the eyes and mouth and to anyone with "hill and valley" acne scarring.

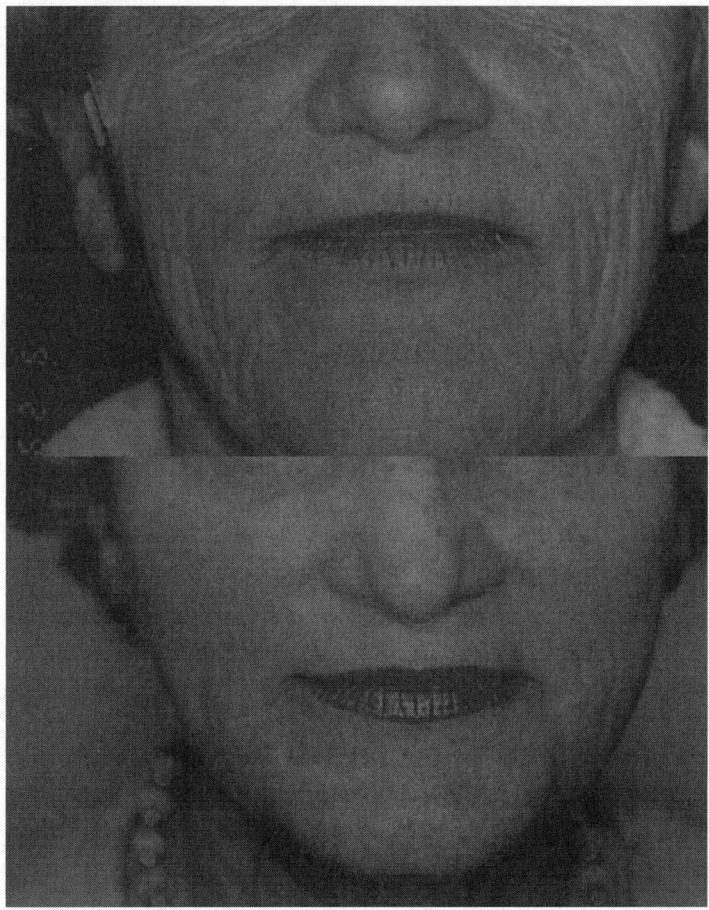

CO_2 laser resurfacing.

How Often: Once.
Cost: $1,500 for a localized area; $6,000–$7,000 for the entire face.

Erbium Laser
Background: The Erbium laser penetrates less deeply into the skin than the CO_2, removing the top layer and a smaller amount of the lower layer. Although recovery time, redness, the risk of scarring, and skin discoloration are less than with the carbon dioxide laser, many people may not be satisfied with the results of the Erbium laser. This laser is often used to treat dark circles and crepey skin around the eyes.
Technique: Using the same process as with the carbon dioxide laser, you will be given either a local anaesthetic if the area to be treated is small, or a general anaesthesia, or a local with intravenous sedation if the entire face is undergoing treatment. Protective eyewear must be worn.
Downtime: Five to seven days.
Complications: There will be some redness after the procedure, which will fade within a couple of weeks.
Post-treatment: Sun exposure must be avoided and a sunscreen with an SPF of 60 is to be worn for at least six months afterwards.
Results: There will be some improvement in fine lines and deeper wrinkles, as well as a modest amount of tightening to the skin.
Ideal Candidate: If you have fines lines and wrinkles or require treatment in a localized area, the Erbium laser may be of some benefit. Anyone with "hill and valley" acne scarring can also benefit from the Erbium laser.
Cost: $1,500 for a localized area; $5,000–$7,000 for the entire face.

BLOOD VESSELS
Pulsed Dye Laser – Short Pulse
Background: The pulsed dye laser, which is set at a wavelength of 585 nanometres, is excellent for targeting single blood vessels or small spider veins.

Chapter 5| **Laser Techniques** 67

Technique: No anaesthesia is required for this simple procedure. The problem blood vessel will be targeted by the laser, which will sting as it fires, but the procedure will take only about five minutes to perform. A bruise will immediately appear on the area. Protective eyewear must be worn.

Downtime: None, other than cosmetic. If more than one area is being treated, there may be significant bruising, which can last for seven to ten days.

Complications: There will be bruising in the areas of treatment.

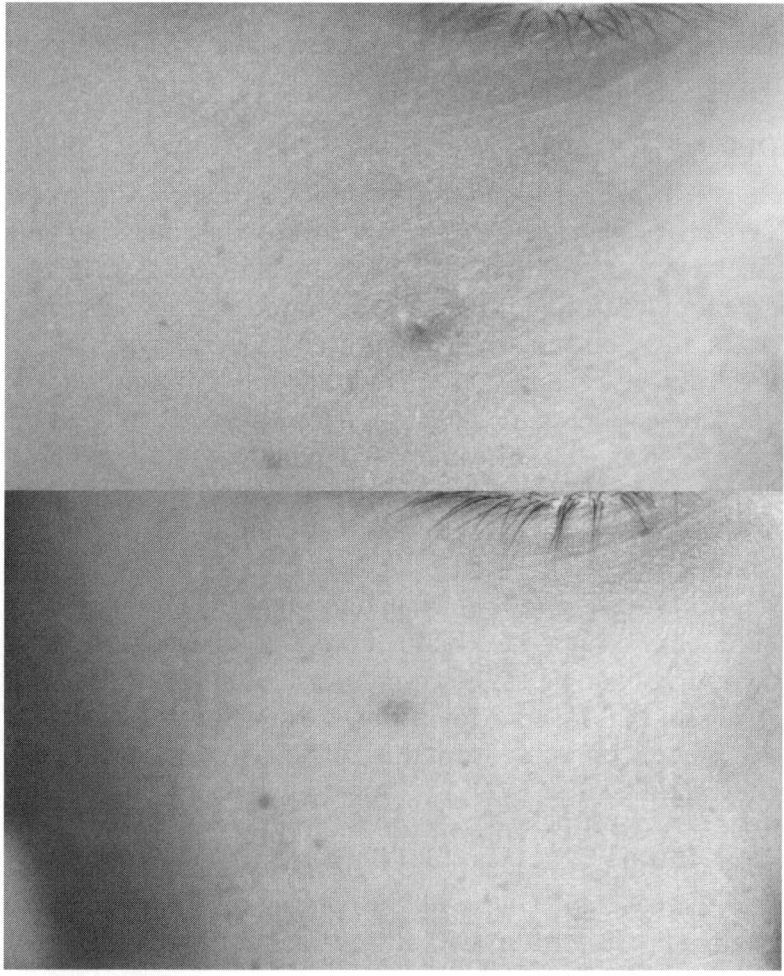

Spider vein improved with PDL

Post-treatment: Cleanse your skin daily in your normal fashion, and apply topical antibiotic cream for three to four days.
Results: This technique is very effective in removing the targeted blood vessels.
Ideal Candidate: Anyone with small broken blood vessels or other small, red lesions on their face will be extremely pleased with the results.
How Often: Once for the treated area. Rarely, a touch-up treatment may be required. Other blood vessels may appear in other areas in the future.
Cost: $150–$500, depending on how many blood vessels have to be targeted.

Pulsed Dye Laser–Long Pulse

Background: A pulsed dye laser–long pulse width has a longer pulse length as compared to the regular PDL and takes a longer time to deliver the energy into the skin. It is an excellent treatment for large areas of redness such as rosacea or any blood-based lesion, with the laser slowly heating the blood vessel and then sealing it. While this method will not bruise the targeted area, there will have to be repeated treatments because the increased pulse length doesn't fully destroy the blood vessel. The most commonly used pulsed dye laser–long wavelength are the V-Star and the V-Beam, which are brand names.
Technique: Taking about a half hour to perform, this procedure requires no anaesthetic. If the V-Beam laser is used, a cooling substance called cryogen will be sprayed onto the skin while the laser is operating. If the V-Star laser is used, cool air will emanate from the tip. Both methods will help alleviate the stinging sensation you will experience as the laser is being fired. You will alternately feel the spray or air, then the hit of the laser, then the spray or air, and so on, during treatment. Even with the cooling substances, expect some mild discomfort with this procedure. Protective eyewear must be worn.

Chapter 5| **Laser Techniques**

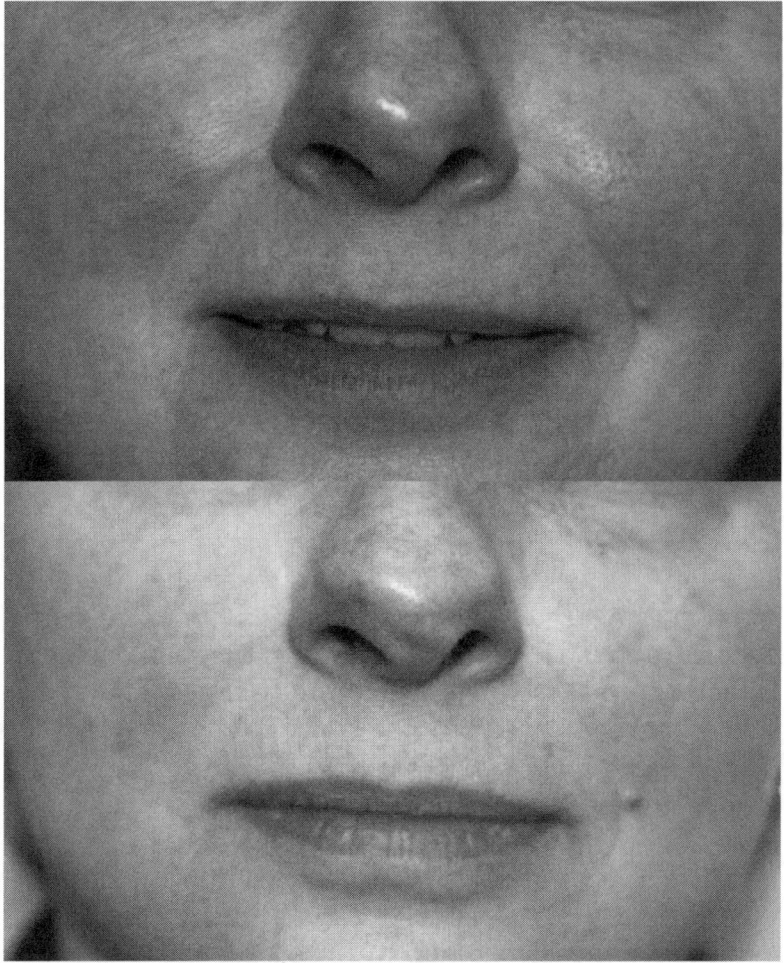

Facial redness diminished with laser

Downtime: None.

Complications: Your skin will be a little red when you leave the doctor's office, but this will disappear after a day or two.

Post-treatment: A sunscreen with an SPF of 60 should be worn for several months after treatment.

Results: There will be no bruising when this form of laser is used; however, you will require multiple treatments before the blood vessels or rosacea fully disappears.

Ideal Candidate: This is an excellent treatment for anyone

with large areas of redness on their skin, who doesn't want the bruising that other methods incur.
How Often: Three to four treatments, spaced at one-month intervals.
Cost: $1,000 (for three treatments). This cost may vary depending on the size of the area being treated and the number of lesions.

Long-Pulse YAG Laser
Background: Operating on a wavelength of 1,064 nanometres, this laser has the capability to treat single large blood vessels (ranging in size from one-half a millimetre to over three millimetres in width) on the face, especially those around the nose and eyes, as well as some superficial leg veins.
Technique: Usually requiring no topical anaesthetic because the lasers have a cooling tip or cooling spray, the procedure will take about a half hour to perform. Expect some pain, however, as the laser fires against your skin. Protective eye shields must be worn.
Downtime: None.
Complications: There is a slight possibility of bruising.
Post-treatment: None.
Results: Excellent results occur after as little as one treatment, with the blood vessel drastically dissipating in size or disappearing all together.
Ideal Candidate: This procedure will benefit anyone with large blood vessels, especially around the nose and eye area.
How Often: One to two times.
Cost: $500 per treatment. The cost will vary on the size of the area being treated.

BROWN/AGE SPOTS
Continuous Wave Laser
Background: The continuous wave laser is sometimes used to treat brown spots on the face, hands, and chest that are typically

Chapter 5| Laser Techniques

caused by sun damage. Set at 532 nanometres, this laser has the potential risk of scarring.

Technique: Usually no anaesthesia is required, although there will be some stinging during the procedure. If you are sensitive to pain, ask your doctor for a topical anaesthetic. Depending on the number of brown spots being treated, the entire procedure should take no longer than a half an hour. Protective eyewear must be worn.

Downtime: Seven to ten days, depending on the area and amount of brown spots being treated.

Complications: There will be blistering and scabbing afterwards, and there may also be a risk of scarring. The area will usually heal in a little redder or whiter before returning to your normal skin colour. There is a possibility that the skin will remain lighter than the surrounding area even after healing.

Post-treatment: You will have to cleanse the treated areas and apply an emollient such as Vaseline. It is important that you protect yourself from the sun afterwards and wear a sunscreen with an SPF of 60, or the areas will heal darker than normal.

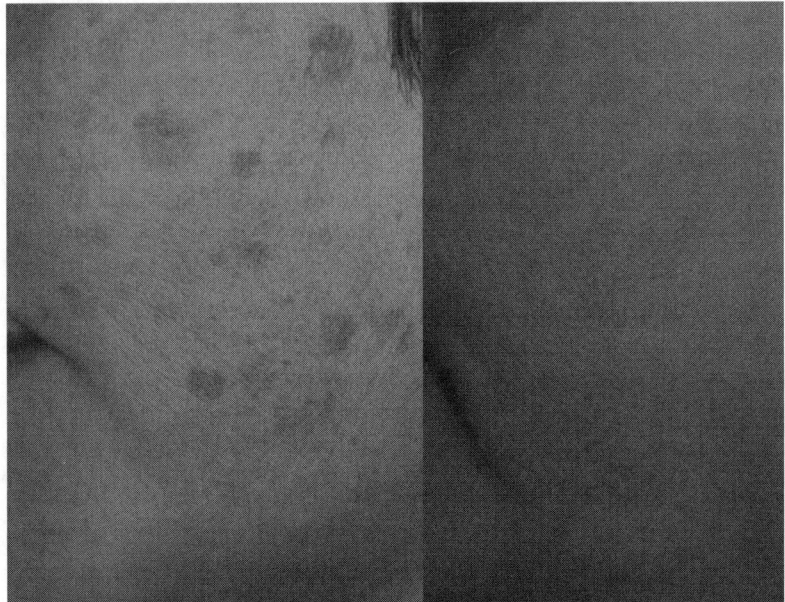

Brown spots removed with Yag laser.

Results: Despite the possible risk of scarring, the continuous wave laser is an effective way to eliminate brown spots anywhere on the body.
Ideal Candidate: This procedure is for someone who has brown spots caused by sun damage. The face, chest, and backs of the hands are the most commonly treated areas. Other types of brown spots such as light brown birthmarks, called café-au-lait marks, also respond well to the continuous wave laser. Brown birth moles that are raised and hairy will not respond to this or any other laser treatment, and should be assessed by a dermatologist prior to any treatment, including electrolysis.
How Often: Once. Over time other brown spots may appear in other areas with continued sun exposure.
Cost: $300–$600 depending on the number of brown spots.

Q-Switched Lasers

Background: There are three types of Q-switched lasers, called Q-switched alexandrite, Q-switched ruby, and the Q-switched Nd:YAG. Even though they are set at different wavelengths, these lasers are all extremely selective when hitting the melanin. Another main advantage in the use of the Q-switched lasers is that there is very little risk of scarring.
Technique: Although no anaesthetic is usually required, there is some discomfort involved with the Q-switched lasers in the form of a stinging sensation when the laser fires against the skin. You may want to ask your doctor for a topically applied cream, or an injection. Depending on the amount of brown spots to be removed, treatment should last no longer than a few minutes. Protective eyewear must be worn.
Downtime: Seven to ten days, depending on the number of brown spots being treated.
Complications: There will be blistering and scabbing of the treated areas. The scabs usually drop off after a week to a week and a half. Sometimes the area will heal in redder or whiter before resuming its normal skin colour. Occasionally, the skin

Chapter 5| **Laser Techniques** 73

may remain lighter in colour than the surrounding area.
Post-treatment: Proper cleansing and application of an emollient such as Vaseline will be required. It is imperative to avoid sun exposure after this treatment since it may cause the treated areas to darken in colour. Application of sunscreen with an SPF 60 should be worn for several weeks afterwards.
Results: Q-switched lasers will effectively remove brown spots anywhere on the body.
Ideal Candidate: For anyone who has brown spots caused by sun exposure, or light brown birthmarks, the Q-switched laser is extremely effective. These lasers, (or any other lasers) will not work on raised, hairy, brown birth moles.
How Often: Once. More brown spots may develop over time on other areas of the body.
Cost: $300–$600, depending on the number of brown spots.

TATTOOS
Q-Switched Lasers
Background: In most cases a combination of the Q-switched lasers should be used on tattoos because of the various colours of the ink that will have to be targeted. The Nd:YAG laser is effective at removing red and black ink, while the Q-switched ruby and alexandrite are good at targeting black and green ink. If you want optimum results, you should choose a doctor's office that is equipped with all of these lasers, since they will be used in conjunction with one another.
Treatment: If the tattoo is cosmetic in nature (permanently inked eyeliner, lipliner, eyebrows), a small area must be tested since the flesh-coloured, rust, or white ink used to dye the skin for the tattoo may immediately turn dark upon laser treatment as the result of a chemical reaction.

A topical anaesthetic may be applied or a local anaesthetic may be used, and the length of time the procedure will take depends on the size of the tattoo being removed. Protective eyewear must be worn.

Downtime: Six to twelve days, depending on the area and the size of the tattoo.
Complications: The treated areas will blister and scab. If the procedure is done on the face or upper body, it will heal much faster than on the legs, which are further away from the heart and its blood supply.
Post-treatment: The area will have to be cleansed and treated with an emollient such as Vaseline or a topical antibiotic ointment during the scabbing stage of healing.
Results: Using a combination of the Q-switched lasers, tattoos can be effectively removed with multiple treatments.
Ideal Candidate: Anyone with a professional tattoo (done by a tattoo artist) or an amateur tattoo (done by piercing one's own skin and injecting India ink), will benefit from the procedure. Those with cosmetic tattoos may also see results, but they must be tested first to ensure a chemical reaction doesn't occur that darkens the pigment.
How Often: Five to eight treatments for amateur tattoos. Six to twenty treatments for professional and cosmetic tattoos.
Cost: $400–$1,000 for first treatment, depending on the size, colour, and complexity of the tattoo. Subsequent treatments will cost less.

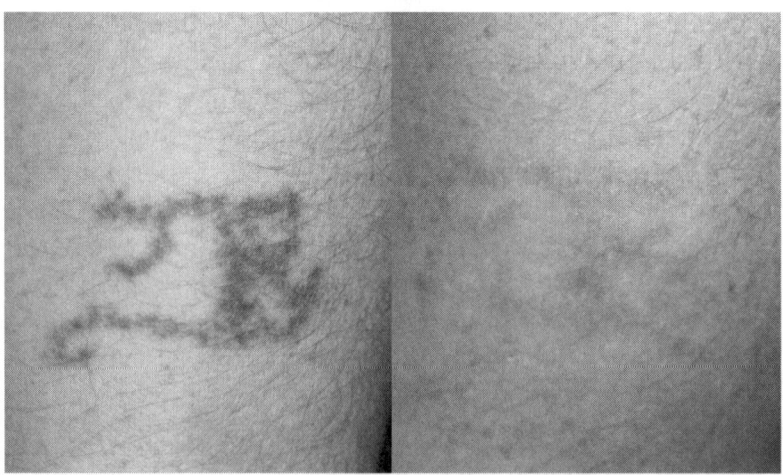

Tattoo removed with laser.

Chapter 5| **Laser Techniques** 75

HAIR REMOVAL
Long-Pulsed Alexandrite, YAG and Diode Lasers

Background: Since the mid-1990s, lasers have been routinely used to remove unwanted hair from the body. Most frequently targeting the hair on the face, under the arms, and on the legs, laser treatment is very effective. The most common types of lasers being used in this procedure are the long-pulsed alexandrite (e.g., the GentleLASE, set at 755 nanometres),

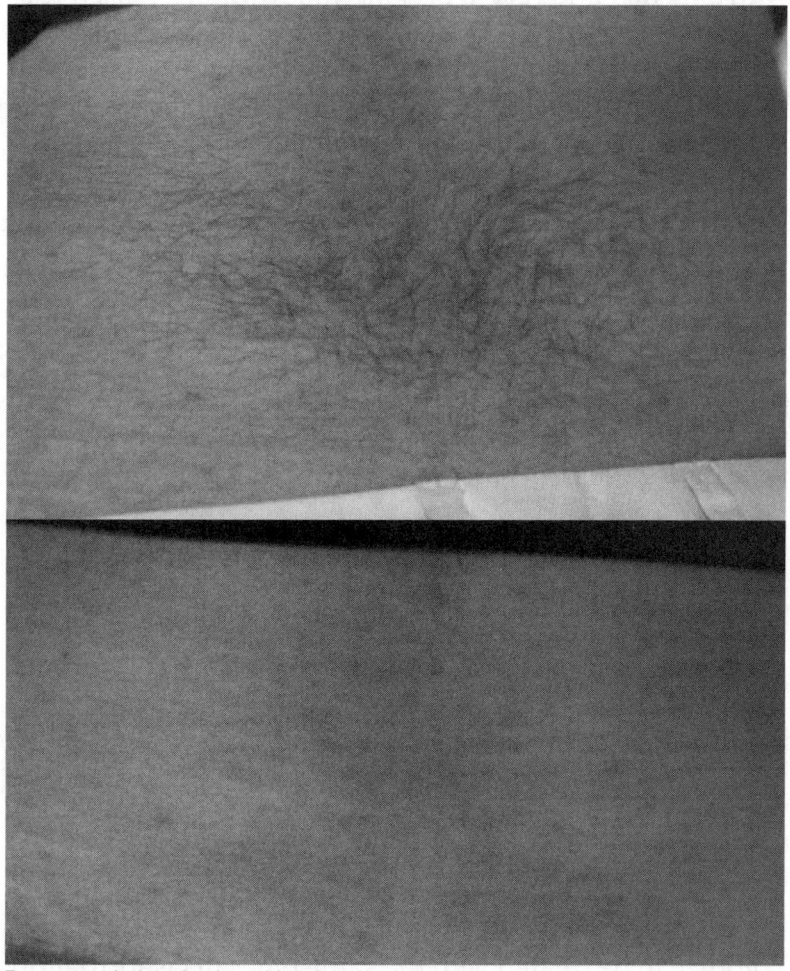

Permanent hair reduction with a laser.

the diode (e.g., LightSheer, set at 800 nanometres), and the long-pulsed YAG (e.g., the CoolGlide, or Sciton, set at 1064 nanometres). Because the colour of the skin is mainly concentrated in the hair follicles, the colour of the follicle will absorb the laser light, heat up the follicle and destroy it.

Laser hair removal will only be effective on those persons with dark hair ranging from medium brown to black. It will not work on people with blonde, grey or red hair. The long-pulsed alexandrite and diode lasers will be used on people with dark hair and very light skin, while the long-pulsed YAG is used on those with dark hair and any skin colour.

Technique: Little to no anaesthesia is required when using any of these lasers because all are equipped with either a cold air/ spray or cooling tip, which will help to alleviate any discomfort you may have when the laser fires. Depending on the size of the area being treated, the procedure will take anywhere from a few minutes to an hour. Protective eyewear must be worn.

Downtime: None.

Complications: The treated area may be a little red and swollen afterwards, but this will subside over a short period of time.

Post-treatment: None.

Results: Although the hair follicles will never be completely eradicated, they will be significantly reduced.

Ideal Candidate: If you have dark hair, you can benefit from laser hair removal. Blonde, grey and red-headed persons are not candidates for this procedure.

How Often: Minimum of five treatments.

Cost: $300 per treatment for smaller areas such as the upper lip or bikini line; $1,000–$2,000 per treatment for larger areas such as the legs or back.

STRETCH MARKS
Pulsed Dye Laser–Long Pulse

Background: There are two types of stretch marks. The first category are the fresh, red marks, which because of their colour, can be treated with the same types of lasers that rid the skin of blood vessels, such as the V-Star or V-Beam. The second type of stretch mark are the thin white or silver marks that have usually been on the body for a long time. Although an Excimer laser set at 308 nanometres may bring some colour back into a white stretch mark, causing it to blend in with the surrounding skin, success rates aren't all that high. Currently, there is nothing that can rid the body of this type of stretch mark; however, there is some evidence to suggest that Thermage (see Chapter 3, "Nonablative Resurfacing of the Skin") may improve the appearance.

Technique: No anaesthesia is required because of the cold air or cold spray that will emanate from the laser. The duration of treatment will depend on the amount and length of stretch marks. Protective eyewear must be worn.

Downtime: None.

Complications: None.

Post-treatment: A sunscreen with an SPF of 60 should be worn during treatment and for several months afterwards.

Results: After multiple treatments, the red stretch mark will fade to a silvery, white line.

Ideal Candidate: This treatment is good for anyone who has fresh, red stretch marks. If you have stretch marks that are thin and silvery in colour, this laser treatment will not work.

How Often: Three to four treatments.

Cost: $300–$700 per treatment.

ACNE SCARS
Pulsed Dye Laser–Long Pulse

Background: Red acne scars respond well to the same lasers that treat broken blood vessels. Typically, the V-Star or the V-Beam lasers are used in this procedure.

Technique: No anaesthesia is required since both lasers are equipped with either a cooling spray or air. Depending on the area being treated, your treatment should last for no longer than half an hour. Protective eye shields must be worn.

Downtime: None.

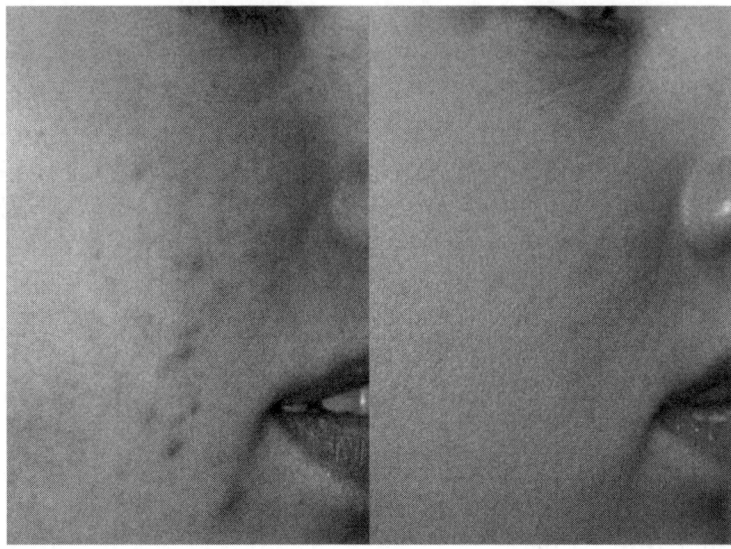

Acne scars improved with a V-Star laser.

Complications: None.
Post-treatment: A sunscreen with an SPF of 60 should be worn during treatment and for several months afterwards.
Results: Although the acne scar will not be removed, the redness will dissipate after multiple treatments, and the appearance of the scar will be less noticeable.
Ideal Candidate: This treatment will work well on anyone who has red acne scars.
How Often: Three to four treatments.
Cost: $400 per treatment.

CO_2/Erbium Lasers

Background: When there is a rolling depression in the skin called "hill and valley" acne, the CO_2 or Erbium lasers work best through their ablative action, which will remove the top layer of skin, heat up the collagen, and force it to tighten.
Technique: For a small area of skin, a local anaesthetic may be used, but for larger areas, such as the entire face, you will be given a general anaesthesia or a local with intravenous

sedation. To treat the entire face, it will take approximately an hour, and protective eyewear must be worn.
Downtime: Five to twelve days (a longer recovery time is required with the CO_2 laser).
Complications: If the CO_2 laser is being used, there will be prolonged redness afterwards, oozing, and possible risk of scarring. If the Erbium laser is used, there will be redness afterwards, however the healing time and risk of scarring will be less.
Post-treatment: The treated areas must be cleansed and dressed properly and your doctor will prescribe exact treatment. Sun exposure must be avoided afterwards and a sunscreen with an SPF of 60 should be worn for several months.
Results: The CO_2 laser offers approximately a 40 percent rate of improvement in repairing "hill and valley" acne scars, while the Erbium laser will have a less than 40 percent improvement, since it does not penetrate the skin as deeply.
Ideal Candidate: These laser treatments will benefit someone with severe, rolling depressions in the skin caused by acne scarring. They will not help diminish the appearance of "ice pick" (deep pits) acne.
How Often: Once.
Cost: $800–$4,000 depending on the size of the area.

Smoothbeam Laser

Background: Used to treat both ice pick scars and "hill and valley" acne scars, the nonablative Smoothbeam laser has demonstrated some success. Although improvement in the acne scarring is not dramatic, this laser does have the ability to decrease the size of the pores and oil glands, as well as stimulate collagen, which will offer some visual refinement of the skin. Combining the Smoothbeam laser with Thermage (see Chapter 3, "Nonablative Resurfacing of the Skin") achieves excellent results.
Technique: A topical anaesthetic will be applied to the area being treated, and there will be a stinging sensation when

the laser fires. The procedure should take under half an hour, and protective eyewear must be worn.

Downtime: Approximately 24 hours; you should be able to return to your normal routine the next day.

Complications: You may be a little red after the procedure, and you could have some pigmentation changes, but they will quickly fade. There is a low risk of scarring with the Smoothbeam laser.

Post-treatment: Avoid sun exposure after treatment and wear a suncreen with an SPF of 25 or higher after treatments.

Results: There will be a noticeable improvement in the acne scars after multiple treatments.

Ideal Candidate: If you have ice pick scars or a rolling depression in the skin caused by "hill and valley" acne scars, you are a good candidate for this procedure. Those with red acne scars will not benefit from the Smoothbeam laser.

How Often: Up to six treatments.

Cost: $300–$500 per treatment.

KELOID SCARS
Pulsed Dye Laser–Long Pulse

Background: Typically caused by an injury or surgery, keloid scars are thick, red, and raised, and are occasionally itchy and sore. Using a combination of laser therapy, cortisone, and silicone gel, most keloid scars can be improved after several treatments. Because of the colour of the scar, the most suitable laser would be one that targets red, such as the pulse dye. New scars respond better to laser treatment than old scars.

Technique: You will not require anaesthetic for the procedure, since the lasers are equipped with a cooling spray or air. The length of treatment will depend on the size of the scar, but will most likely take under half an hour. Protective eyewear must be worn.

Downtime: None.

Complications: None.

Chapter 5| **Laser Techniques** 81

Post-treatment: You will require cortisone injections to thin the skin, and your exact treatment will be prescribed by your doctor. Wear a sunscreen with an SPF of 60 during treatment and for several months afterwards.
Results: The scar will decrease after multiple treatments.
Ideal Candidate: If you have a large, raised, red scar caused by injury or surgery, you will benefit from the laser and cortisone treatment.
How Often: Eight to nine treatments.
Cost: $400 per treatment.

LEG VEINS
Long-Pulse Nd:YAG

Background: There are several ways to treat leg veins and the most common options include tying off larger veins and/or sclerotherapy, which involves injecting the superficial or spider veins with a solution (see Chapter 7, "Leg Veins"). Currently, many dermatologists are targeting these same tiny legs veins with a long-pulse Nd:YAG laser such as the CoolGlide or Sciton.
Technique: Taking about a half hour to perform, the superficial blood vessels in your legs will be hit with the laser. Although this procedure is somewhat painful, the sting will be alleviated by the cooling tip or spray. Protective eyewear must be worn.
Downtime: None.
Complications: There may be some bruising on the treated areas, but this will fade within a few days to weeks. Hyperpigmentation may also occur and last months.
Post-treatment: None.
Results: Superficial spider veins in the legs will disappear in as little as one treatment.
Ideal Candidate: This procedure may benefit someone with tiny broken blood vessels in the legs.
How Often: One to two times.
Cost: $500 per treatment.

Endovenous Laser Therapy

Background: The relatively new technique called endovenous (in the vein) laser therapy has proven successful at removing large leg or varicose veins and is a good alternative to the traditional stripping of these veins. The procedure involves threading a laser into the patient's blood vessel and shooting light into the vein from the inside.

Technique: You will be given a local anaesthesia prior to the treatment. First, a small incision will be made in your leg, where a laser fibre will be inserted into the greater saphenous vein, which runs from the knee to the groin. Then the laser light will be delivered into the vein, causing it to collapse and seal shut. The entire procedure should take no more than an hour to perform.

Downtime: 24 hours, with most patients returning to normal activity the next day.

Complications: There will most likely be bruising after treatment. There is also a slight possibility of skin burn, paresthesia (numbness or tingling sensations), and in rare cases, deep vein thrombosis (blood clots).

Post-treatment: Compression stockings must be worn for up to a week after treatment.

Results: The success rate is very high in removing deep varicose veins with minimal pain and discomfort. There are also excellent long-term results, with 98 percent of the veins remaining shut after three years.

Ideal Candidate: This procedure would appeal to someone with deep leg veins who does not want to undergo the pain and longer recovery time of the traditional stripping technique.

How Often: Once.

Cost: $3000–$6000

Chapter 5 | **Laser Techniques** 83

MOST COMMONLY ASKED QUESTIONS

Question: How can I treat rosacea and broken blood vessels on my cheeks and on and around my nose?

Answer: These conditions can be treated with a combination of a long-pulse dye laser together with a long-pulse YAG laser. Although it will sometimes require three to four sessions, there is little to no downtime involved. Another option would be a series of intense pulse light photo facials used with Levulan (see Chapter 3, "Nonablative Resurfacing of the Skin").

Question: What is the best way to remove a single, large brown spot?

Answer: Such a spot can easily be treated with a laser. Although the procedure will result in some scabbing, the area will heal without any significant colour change.

Question: I have a multicoloured tattoo and was wondering if laser removal is effective?

Answer: It will depend on the colours of the tattoo. Red and black ink will usually respond well to a Q-switched Nd:Yag laser, while most green coloured tattoos can be effectively removed with a Q-switched alexandrite laser. As a whole, approximately 70 percent of patients will have good results, with most of the tattoo cleared and minimal scarring. However, it is important to note that removal will require several sessions and that some tattoos will not clear totally. It is best to go to a clinic with both a Q-switched Nd:Yag and either a Q-switched alexandrite or Q-switched ruby laser.

Question: I have blonde hair and am considering laser hair removal. How effective will it be?

Answer: Laser hair removal is not an effective treatment if you have blonde, red, or grey hair. Typically, laser hair removal works best on those persons with light skin and dark brown or black hair. If you have very dark skin, it is important that your doctor use a long-pulsed YAG system to remove your hair.

Question: I have had multiple pregnancies and as a result, have large, red stretch marks. Is there any way to get rid of them?

Answer: Stretch marks are very difficult to treat. Although many topical creams have been advertised as a treatment, they are typically ineffective. The pulsed dye laser will improve the color of the stretch mark, but there will still be a white, silvery mark remaining. For the white, silvery marks, you may want to try Thermage (see Chapter 3, "Nonablative Resurfacing of the Skin"). The stretch mark will not disappear, but there is some evidence to suggest that it may be improved.

Question: Is there a laser treatment for deep wrinkles in my forehead, around my eyes, cheeks and lips?

Answer: Deep wrinkles will only respond well to a resurfacing procedure using the Erbium laser or the carbon dioxide laser. While the Erbium laser has less downtime and few side effects, it will be less effective than the carbon dioxide laser, which significantly improves wrinkles. However, there is a considerable recovery period, followed by complications such as prolonged redness and loss of pigment in some patients. Treatment mayb be combined with Botox for best results.

Question: What can I do for large pores on my forehead, nose and cheeks?

Answer: While vitamin A may help clean out the pores, it will not reduce their size. Other types of creams will temporarily improve the look of the surrounding skin, making the pore appear smaller until the cream is washed off. The only effective way to reduce the pore size is through laser treatment utilizing the Smoothbeam.

Question: I have "spider veins" in my legs. Can a laser remove them?

Answer: Laser treatment is most effective in treating large, deep leg veins through the endovenous technique. Occasionally, a laser may be useful for some smaller leg veins, but it is really not very effective. Not only is it expensive, but you may also get side effects such as pigmentation changes. The best way to treat superficial leg veins is with sclerotherapy (see Chapter 7, "Leg Veins").

Chapter 5| **Laser Techniques** 85

Question: Can ingrown hairs be treated with a laser?
Answer: Because dark hair absorbs the laser light, which destroys the hair at the root, ingrown hairs can be treated with a laser. The procedure can also limit the risk of future regrowth.

Chapter 6

Wrinkles

Wrinkles are probably the number one reason why women flock to their dermatologists' offices in droves. Seeming to pop up overnight, these lines and furrows can make our faces appear tired, angry, tense, and old. Makeup becomes more difficult to apply, and what used to be a relatively simple procedure takes longer and longer each morning as we attempt to camouflage the ravages of mother nature. Powders, foundations, and concealers settle into the fine and deeper lines on our faces, often making us appear even older than we are. Eyeshadow becomes a nightmare to apply, and anyone over the age of fifty is well acquainted with the frustration of having lipstick creep into the vertical lines around the mouth.

    We already know the main cause of wrinkles—intrinsic aging, gravity, environmental pollutants, and the sun. Called static wrinkles, we can't even avoid them when we're sleeping because as we get older and lose the elasticity in our skin, wrinkles will form simply by the pressure from putting our faces against a pillow. But there is also a second type of wrinkle, which is caused by habitual movement. Known as dynamic wrinkles, they are more commonly seen on the forehead, between the eyebrows, around the eyes and lips, and down the sides of the nose.

Both static and dynamic wrinkles can be treated, but first the dermatologist must determine the underlying cause and then treat the cause. Static wrinkles will usually call for some type of filler, such as collagen, fat, or hyaluronic acid to plump and soften them, while dynamic wrinkles require Botox injections, which will stop the movement that originally produced the wrinkle.

Following are some of the more common and preferred ways to treat wrinkles because they involve minimal pain and downtime.

COLLAGEN

Background: Collagen is one of the main components that makes up our skin structure, and as we age, it degenerates, causing deep lines and wrinkles to form. In an attempt to replace our natural collagen, scientists began to look at the possibility of injecting the facial lines with a close substitute. The first legally approved collagen filler came from cows, and is generally known as bovine collagen, with the trade names of Zyplast and Zyderm. Many patients have an allergic reaction to bovine collagen, and skin tests must be performed before treatment. There is also a second type of collagen, which is derived from a human culture (fetal foreskin), with the trade names of CosmoDerm and CosmoPlast. Because human collagen originates from an isolated cell culture, allergic reaction is extremely rare and patients need not be pretested.

Both forms of collagen are most often used to treat the folds that run vertically down the sides of the nose to the mouth (called the nasolabial folds). It can also be used on the vertical lines that form around the mouth, to plump the lips, which tend to lose their fullness as we age, and sometimes on the 11-shaped furrow that forms between the eyebrows, known as the glabellar lines. (The medical term for augmenting the lips with collagen or any other type of filler is *cheiloplasty*.) While collagen can be useful in all these areas, it is not recommended for treating the skin around the eyes or on the forehead because it tends to be bumpy in consistency and would be noticeable in these thinner-skinned areas.

Technique: If bovine collagen is being used, you must undergo a series of testing for allergic response. The first test will take place four weeks prior to treatment, and then another test will be performed two weeks before treatment. With either type of collagen, a local anaesthetic will be applied topically about an hour before the procedure. The collagen is injected into the desired areas with a needle. Expect some discomfort during the process, which usually takes about fifteen minutes to complete.

Downtime: Little to none.

Complications: There will be some redness and swelling immediately after the procedure that may last for several hours. Although unusual, some redness may last for months afterwards. Any bruising that occurs from the injections should fade within days. Even with pretesting, one to three percent of patients may still develop a severe reaction to bovine collagen, and an even smaller number will also have a reaction to the human collagen. Collagen tends to have a bumpy texture, and small lumps can often be felt and seen in the areas that have been injected.

Post-treatment: Cold packs should be applied to the injected areas to counteract redness and swelling. If the area is bumpy, it should be gently massaged. In rare cases, the bumps (especially in the lip area) will have to be surgically removed.

Results: The lines and wrinkles will diminish in appearance as the skin is plumped or filled with the collagen; however, the effect is temporary. Your own natural collagen may also be stimulated by the filler and begin to regenerate.

Ideal Candidate: This procedure may be of benefit for those with deep lines running down the sides of the nose, vertical lines around the mouth, and lips that have shrunk or thinned out in size.

How Often: Every three to four months.

Cost: $200–$1,500 per treatment, depending on the area being treated. Half a syringe costs $250 and is usually enough to treat fine lines. A full syringe costs $500, and three syringes will be required for the nasolabial folds.

HYALURONIC ACID

Background: Hyaluronic acid is the natural fluid our skin sits in, and its derivatives are fast becoming the preferred choice of dermatologists when using soft-tissue fillers to diminish the appearance of wrinkles. Because hyaluronic acid is identical in all species, it can be taken from different sources and injected just beneath the skin with little risk of complication. First developed in Europe in the 1990s, the most commonly used hyaluronic acids, such as Restylane, Perlane, and Juvederm (trade names), are created in a laboratory from a bacterial culture. Being nonanimal in nature, they provide an excellent alternative to collagen, and require no pretesting. Another type of hyaluronic acid is called Hylaform. Because it is derived from a rooster's comb, there is the possibility of allergic reactions to those with animal-related sensitivities.

Injected into the lips, lip lines, crow's feet, nasolabial folds, and glabellar lines, in the form of a clear gel, the hyaluronic acid will bear and bind water, much like our own hyaluronic acid does. Over time, the gel breaks down, is absorbed by the body and after several months is totally eliminated.

Aside from the source related variation, the filler gels differ primarily in their concentration levels. The higher the concentration, the longer they will last. Following are some of the most popular hyaluronic acids and what they are used to treat.

Chapter 6| **Wrinkles**   91

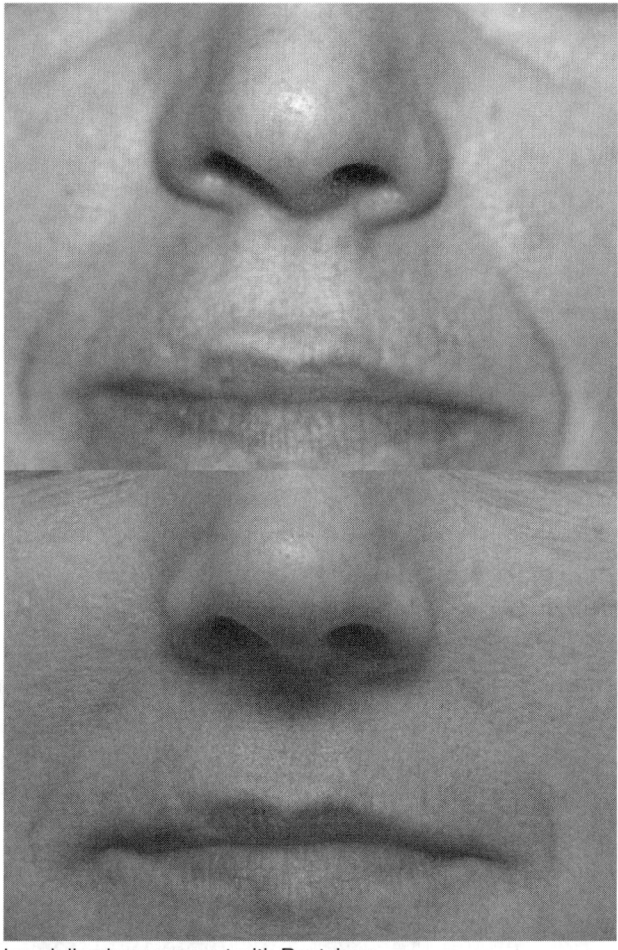

Laugh line improvement with Restylane.

Trade Name	**Used to Treat**
Hylaform Fine Lines	Fine lines
Hylaform Plus	Deeper wrinkles and folds
Restylane Fine Lines	Fine lines
Restylane	Medium lines and wrinkles
Perlane	Deep wrinkles and folds
Juvederm 18	Fine lines
Juvederm 24	Medium lines and wrinkles
Juvederm 30	Deep wrinkles and folds

Technique: About an hour before the procedure, a topical anaesthetic will be applied to numb the area. This is especially important if the lips are to be treated, since they tend to be more sensitive to pain. Your lines, wrinkles, or folds will be injected with the hyaluronic acid of choice, with the procedure taking approximately fifteen minutes to perform. Expect some discomfort, especially with the higher concentrations of filler, since a larger needle must be used.

Downtime: None.

Complications: Immediately after the procedure there will be some redness and possible swelling, which can last for several days. Bruising may occur in the areas of injection, but the discoloration will fade within a few days. Small bumps under the skin may also be apparent. Allergic reaction to Hylaform is a possible risk, while reaction to the hyaluronic acid created from bacterial cultures is rare.

Post-treatment: Cold packs should be applied to the areas that are red and swollen. If there are noticeable bumps under the skin, they should be gently massaged for a few days.

Results: Nasolabial and glabellar lines will diminish dramatically, as will the fine lines around the mouth. Lips will appear fuller and smoother. The injections may also stimulate your own natural collagen.

Ideal Candidate: Hyaluronic acid injectable fillers are best suited to those who have deep folds at the sides of the nose, frown lines between the eyebrows, or vertical lines around the mouth. Anyone whose lips have decreased in size because of aging will also benefit from the injections.

How Often: Every three to six months to a year.

Cost: $250–$1,500 depending on the area being treated. A half syringe costs $250 and would be sufficient to treat some of the fine lines around the mouth. A full syringe costs $450 and would be enough to inject the lips. Nasolabial folds and glabellar lines would require two to three full syringes.

ARTECOLL

Background: Considered to be one of the longest-lasting implants, Artecoll is a mixture of bovine collagen and microscopic PMMA beads. PMMA (polymethyl methacrylate) is a biocompatible polymer that has been used in medicine since the 1930s. Once injected into the wrinkle or fold, the beads become enmeshed with your own collagen, and within a few months your natural collagen will begin to regenerate, dramatically reducing the wrinkles. Best used in the treatment of the deep nasal folds, it can also be used in the lips, and will generally last for over five years. Because it is made with bovine collagen, pretesting for allergies is mandatory.

Another permanent type filler is called DermaLive or DermaDeep, which is a mixture of hyaluronic acid and acrylic hydrogel particles. Working in much the same way as Artecoll, DermaLive and DermaDeep will also endure for many years. Other long-lasting fillers that your doctor may use are Radiance, Sculptra, and silicone.

Technique: If Artecoll is being used, a pretest will usually be performed two weeks before the procedure to check for allergies. Although Artecoll is also mixed with lidocaine, which is an anaesthetic, you will also require a topical anaesthetic or an injection for either product. Even then, expect some discomfort since the needle used for these treatments is larger. The injection process should take no longer than fifteen minutes.

Downtime: None.

Complications: There will be some immediate redness and swelling, and because the needle that is used for the injections is larger, there may be some bruising. Bumps in the injected areas are common, and in some cases, they may have to be surgically removed or treated with cortisone. Because the implant is long lasting, most doctors will recommend a temporary filler first, such as Restylane. If you like the results, then a permanent filler can be used once the Restylane has broken down.

Post-treatment: Cold packs should be applied to the areas to treat the redness and swelling. Any bumpy areas should be gently massaged.

Results: After two to three months, your deep lines and wrinkles will have dramatically reduced. As your own collagen continues to rebuild, your face will appear younger with fewer lines, wrinkles, and folds.

Ideal Candidate: If you have deep lines, wrinkles, and folds or thinning lips and have tried a temporary filler with success, you may benefit from the long-lasting implant.

How Often: One to two times, depending on the desired effect and the area being treated.

Cost: $750–$6,000. A syringe costs $750. To inject the nasal folds or the lips, two to four syringes are required for each area.

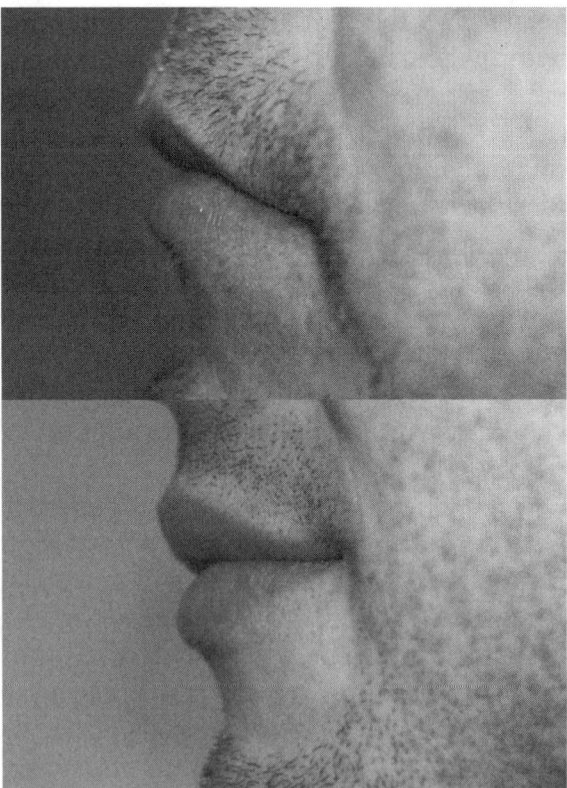

Lip enhancement with Artecoll.

FAT TRANSPLANTATION

Background: Used in conjunction with liposuction, and often done at the same time as a facelift (see Chapter 8, "Face, Brow, and Eye Lifts," and Chapter 10, "Body Contouring"), taking fat from an area of your body and injecting it into another area is a common way to permanently fill in deep folds and wrinkles. It is also routinely used by plastic surgeons to contour parts of the face, such as the cheek area, and to plump up the lips or the back of the hands. While easy to obtain, the downside in using fat is that after it has been injected into the site, there can be up to a 50 percent loss of the substance, and a repeated procedure will most likely be necessary after a year.

Technique: If you are having a full liposuction procedure, the doctor can use some of the removed fat for injection purposes. If you do not require this procedure, the doctor will perform a minimal amount of liposuction utilizing a small incision, usually in the abdomen or buttocks, then using a syringe to draw out the fat. Using a larger needle than the temporary fillers, the fat will then be injected into the various areas of the face or hands.

Downtime: Seven days (mainly for cosmetic reasons since there will be swelling and bruising).

Complications: There will be the usual risks associated with liposuction (see Chapter 10). Expect swelling, bruising, and some minor discomfort for about a week. Other than the up to 50 percent loss of the fat during the first year, the results of this procedure are permanent. Therefore, most doctors will recommend trying a temporary filler first, especially in the lips, before ultimately deciding on fat transplants.

Post-treatment: Ice can be applied to counteract the swelling and bruising and a mild pain medication such as Tylenol can be taken.

Results: Deep folds along the side of the nose can be dramatically improved. Lips and the backs of the hands will be plumper and more youthful looking. If used in the cheek area

(see Chapter 9, "Facial Contouring"), the cheeks will be lifted and more prominent. Because of the thick consistency of the fat, this is not a good treatment for fine lines and wrinkles.
Ideal Candidate: If you have tried a temporary filler in the lips or nasolabial folds and have been pleased with the results, you may want to have this procedure. Fat transfers will also be of benefit if you want your cheeks lifted or the backs of your hands to appear plumper and less crepey.
How Often: Twice, since most fat injections will require a second operation after a year.
Cost: $500. If done with a full liposuction procedure, the cost will be higher than if done alone (see Chapter 10, "Body Contouring").

BOTOX

Background: The botulinum toxin was first isolated in Belgium after several people became ill at a picnic, and eventually the medical community was using it to treat muscle disorders around the eye and in the neck. In the early 1990s, a Canadian ophthalmologist by the name of Jean Carruthers was using the toxin to treat misalignment of the eyes in her patients and noticed the smoothing effect it was having on wrinkles around the sites of injection. After another decade of research, Botox was released on the market as a cosmetic treatment for fine lines and wrinkles on the face.

Derived from a purified protein, Botox prevents muscles from contracting by blocking the nerve signals from the nerve to the muscle. By relaxing the muscles that cause wrinkles, the continued use of this injection will soften existing lines and help deter future wrinkles from forming.

Since its availability in the marketplace, millions of injections of Botox have been given, making the treatment the most common of all cosmetic procedures. It is even now used to treat children as young as two years of age who have cerebral palsy, improving their muscle movement.

One of the main myths surrounding this breakthrough cosmetic treatment is that it will paralyze the injected muscles, not allowing any expressions to show. Naysayers would have you believe that the face will freeze and appear unanimated. The truth is that if Botox is injected properly, the surrounding muscles will relax, and the effects will be subtle and natural. It is only when Botox is used by an inexperienced person that horror stories can happen. Too much Botox injected in the wrong places can not only create a frozen and tight look, it may also trigger medical problems such as a droopy eyelid. If injected incorrectly, it can also cause your eyebrows and forehead to drop. Therefore, you should see only a qualified medical professional if you are thinking of getting this procedure.

Most commonly used on the forehead grooves, the glabellar lines between the eyebrows, and on crow's feet around the eyes, Botox is sometimes also used on the lines around the lips, the vertical and horizontal neckline bands that run from the neck to the chin, and can even be used on the corners of the mouth to turn it up (mesolabial or marionette lines). You must be cautioned, however, that too high a dose on the lip line can affect the way you speak afterwards. If you are older and have loose skin directly under the eye, you should also be wary about receiving injections in that area. Besides needing those muscles to push fluids away from the eye, the injection may cause the lower eyelid to turn out, creating an unnatural look.

Technique: No anaesthetic will be required for this ten to fifteen minute procedure, since the needles used are extremely fine. The underlying muscle where the wrinkle appears will be injected. If done by a qualified doctor, there should be minimum or no pain.

Downtime: None.

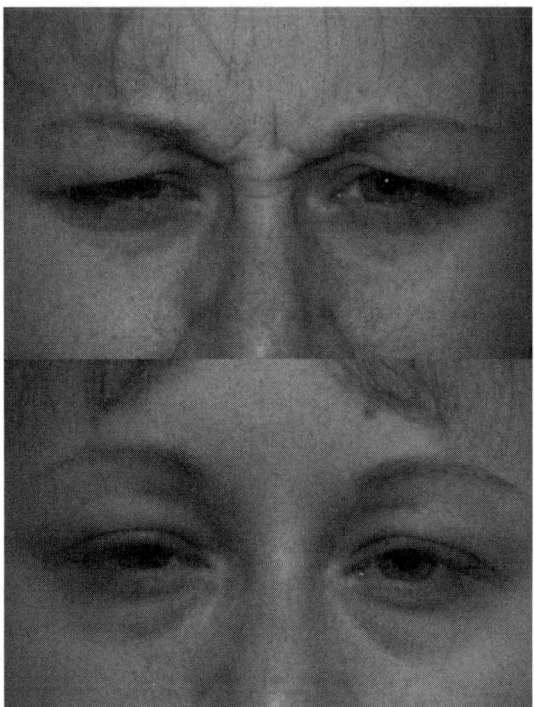

Frown lines corrected with Botox.

Complications: There may be mild, temporary bruising in the areas injected. If the forehead is being treated, you may experience a slight headache immediately afterwards, which can last for a few hours. Because Botox is a medicine, it must be prescribed and performed by a qualified physician. If not, complications can be severe and varied as outlined above. Even in the hands of an experienced doctor, brow and eyelid droop can happen, but this is a rare occurrence. If the brow droops, the patient will have to wait three to four months until the effects of the Botox have worn off. If the eyelid droops, Ipodine drops will be prescribed. These drops will stimulate a muscle in the eyelid to contract and lift the eyelid.

Post-treatment: None.

Results: If injected properly, Botox has the capability to soften lines and wrinkles on the face. The most dramatic changes will be in the forehead, which will appear smooth

Chapter 6| **Wrinkles**

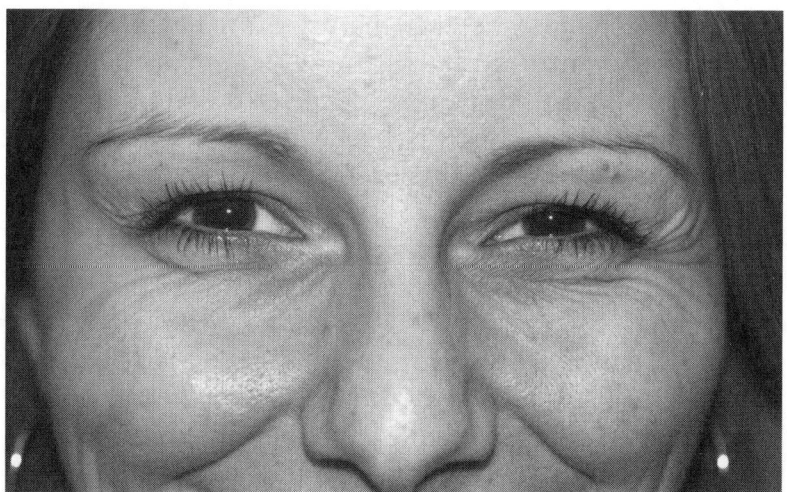

Crow's feet corrected with Botox: one side treated only.

and wrinkle-free and in the area between the brow, where the "11 line" will diminish in appearance. Crow's feet at the outer corners of the eyes will also be less apparent.

Ideal Candidate: Botox is for anyone who would like to appear more rested and relaxed by softening the lines and wrinkles on their forehead, brow area, and around the eyes. It is also a good treatment if you have vertical lines around the lips, or would like to have the corners of your mouth turn upward.

How Often: Once every three to five months. However, the more often an area is treated, the less often it seems to be needed.

Cost: $300–$600. Botox is priced by the unit and an average unit price is between $10 and $11. One area of treatment, such as around the eyes or between the brow, will take thirty units. To inject the forehead, brow, and around the eyes would require sixty units.

MOST COMMONLY ASKED QUESTIONS

Question: No matter how happy and well-rested I am, the older I get, I seem to look tired and angry. What's causing this and what can I do about it?

Answer: This "look" has taken many years to become etched on your face and is caused by the constant contracting of your forehead muscles. These deep furrows tend to make us appear tired or upset. The best way to treat them is with Botox. If the furrows still persist, then they can be filled with a substance such as Restylane or Artecoll.

Question: I used to be a smoker and now have deep lines around my mouth, which my lipstick tends to bleed into. What can I do?

Answer: This is a very common problem and has been caused by the continual pursing of the lips. The area can first be treated with low dosages of Botox, then the outline of the lip margin can be filled with a substance such as Restylane. If necessary, a filler substance can also be injected into the lip lines. The other option is to first use Botox, then resurface the lips with a CO_2 laser, or Erbium laser.

Question: I've already had Botox injected around my eyes, but I still have significant wrinkles underneath my lower eyelid. How can this be treated?

Answer: This area is one of the most difficult to treat. If Botox is injected directly under the lower eyelid, it can result in the eyelid drooping or a gross swelling of the skin. Furthermore, fillers are very difficult to inject under the eye. The only option currently available is to resurface the area with either the Erbium, CO_2, or Smoothbeam lasers (see Chapter 5, "Laser Techniques").

Question: What is the difference between a temporary and a permanent filler?

Answer: Temporary fillers such as Restylane last approximately three to six months, depending on the product and the area being treated. Most temporary fillers are made from hyaluronic acid and will totally disappear after a period of time. Permanent fillers, such as Artecoll or Dermalive, tiny beads, and either collagen or hyaluronic acid. The collagen or hyaluronic acid completely disappears in about three to four weeks, however the particles remain in the skin, causing a foreign-body reaction. This works much like a grain of sand caught in an oyster. Your own collagen builds around the beads and creates a permanent correction.

Question: I take herbal supplements. Can this be harmful prior to my injections?

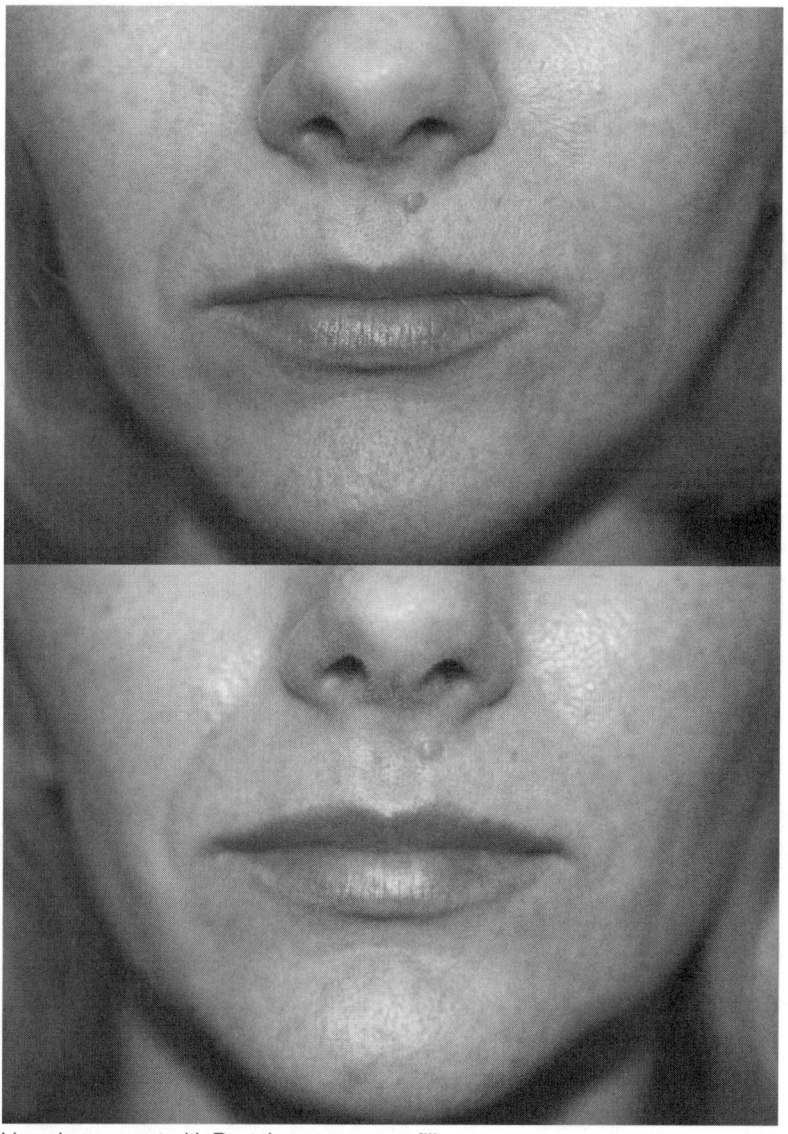

Lip enhancement with Restylane temporary filler.

Answer: Aspirin and anti-inflammatories, such as Advil and Aleve, as well as vitamin E and some herbal supplements increase the risk of bruising and bleeding with any injection such as Botox or fillers. Do not take for 48 hours to a week before your procedure.

Chapter 7

Leg Veins

Unsightly leg veins are an extremely common cosmetic and medical problem, affecting up to 30 percent of women and 18 percent of men. While many of us inherit the underlying causes of leg vein problems from our parents, other factors, such as hormones, pregnancy, standing for long periods of time, physical trauma, aging, and weight gain, can also lead to unattractive leg veins.

Whether inherited or not, all leg vein problems are the result of an impaired return of blood to the heart, called venous insufficiency. The weakened return then causes the pooling of blood in the legs, which causes pressure to build in the deep, superficial, or perforating vein systems. Both spider veins, which are the tiny, broken capillaries that form near the surface of the skin, and the deeper, long ones known as varicose veins, are caused by venous insufficiency involving the superficial veins.

While spider veins are more of a visual annoyance, varicose veins can make your legs ache and sometimes swell. People with serious cases will often experience open skin ulcers and discoloration, and the painful symptoms will force sufferers to seek medical attention.

Aside from utilizing laser therapy (see Chapter 5, "Laser Techniques"), there are several traditional ways of dealing with leg veins.

SCLEROTHERAPY

Background: Sclerotherapy, which involves injecting the leg vein with a sclerosing solution that causes it to collapse, is often the treatment of choice for small spider veins and some varicose veins. The injection process causes inflammation to the vein wall, resulting in the blood vessel closing. Prior to any procedure, your leg veins will be assessed by a physician to determine the most suitable treatment.

Technique: No anaesthetic will be required for this procedure, since the needle that is used is extremely fine. The physician injects the veins with a sclerosing solution, causing most of them to seal off immediately, while an attending nurse covers each area with gauze and tape immediately after the individual injections. Most often, a series of approximately fifteen injections will be given in each leg per session. Expect some discomfort, especially towards the end of the treatment, which should take no longer than thirty minutes.

Downtime: None.

Complications: There may be some temporary hyperpigmentation or discoloration in the areas of injection. In less than 1 percent of cases, the hyperpigmentation is permanent. There is a very rare chance of blood clots, allergic reaction, and skin ulcers.

Post-treatment: If larger veins are injected, you will need to wear compression stockings for a period of time that will be determined by your doctor. Mild exercise such as walking is recommended for a half hour daily for three days after treatment. Avoid heavy exercise, including running or aerobics, for a period of time that will again be determined by your doctor, based on your individual treatment.

Results: Most injected spider veins will disappear almost immediately, while varicose veins may require multiple treatments. Since a limited number of veins can be treated in a single session, several treatments will be required if you are attempting to clear the legs of all veins. Over time, more veins will most likely develop and have to be treated.

Ideal Candidate: If you have several spider veins on your legs that make them appear bruised or blotchy, you will benefit from this treatment. Those with mild to medium varicose veins may also see results.

How Often: Once to treat individual areas of spider veins. More than one treatment will most likely be required to treat varicose veins. To clear the legs of all veins, multiple treatments will be needed and will be determined by the number of veins.

Cost: $60–$100 per session.

ULTRASOUND-GUIDED SCLEROTHERAPY

Background: Ultrasound is used as a method to identify deep veins that cannot be seen, but are causing surface veins to form. Once the vein is targeted, a strong sclerosing chemical will be injected, causing the vein to close.

Technique: After the ultrasound has located the malfunctioning vein, a solution will be injected into the nonvisible vein, which is usually the saphenous vein. A local anaesthetic may be required for the procedure, which can take up to a half hour to perform.

Downtime: None.

Complications: Expect some mild discomfort and inflammation, which can last for several weeks. There is a chance of temporary hyperpigmentation, and a very small risk that it will be permanent. Furthermore, blood that has become trapped between the closed areas may require drainage with a needle.

Post-treatment: Compression stockings will have to be worn for a week after the procedure.

Results: Smaller surface veins that are connected to the targeted larger vein will often lighten or disappear, and further sclerotherapy of smaller spider veins will be enhanced.

Ideal Candidate: If your doctor has determined that problems with your surface veins are caused by deep, hidden veins, you may be a candidate for ultrasound-guided sclerotherapy. This treatment would also be of benefit to those who have undergone endovenous laser therapy (see Chapter 5, "Laser Techniques") as a way to treat any remaining varicose veins.

How Often: Once.

Cost: $250–$500.

VEIN STRIPPING

Background: Traditional vein stripping entails removing the greater saphenous vein that runs from the groin to the knee. Considered an invasive procedure, the operation is performed at a hospital.

Technique: While you are under a general anaesthetic, several incisions will be made into the leg so that a thin rod can be passed up the vein. When this is completed, the rod will be removed, pulling the vein out through the skin in the process.

Downtime: One to two weeks.

Complications: There will be considerable bruising afterwards, which will fade over time. Scarring from the incisions will also occur. Other complications are infrequent but can be severe, including blood clots, damage to the deep veins, and prolonged or permanent numbness.

Post-treatment: Compression stockings must be worn for three weeks after the procedure.

Results: When the greater saphenous vein is removed, other surface veins will lighten or disappear. Results are long-lasting.

Ideal Candidate: If you have large varicose veins and are looking for a time-tested, effective treatment, traditional vein stripping is a definite option.

How Often: Once.
Cost: Considered to be a medical procedure if certain conditions are met, this procedure is usually covered by health insurance.

AMBULATORY PHLEBECTOMY

Background: This procedure is used to remove bulging surface veins and is often confused with vein stripping. The veins are removed through small punctures and the technique is sometimes used in conjunction with ultrasound guided sclerotherapy to close off any deep veins that are causing the problem. It is also an excellent follow up treatment after endovenous laser therapy (see Chapter 5, "Laser Techniques").

Technique: Performed in your doctor's office using a local anaesthetic, small punctures will be made in the leg and the bulging veins will be removed through the openings. Expect some discomfort during the procedure, which should take approximately an hour to an hour and a half to perform.

Downtime: One day.

Complications: There may be minimal and temporary hyperpigmentation. There is also a risk of scarring.

Post-treatment: Compression stockings must be worn for a week following the procedure.

Results: Bulging surface veins will be instantly and permanently removed.

Ideal Candidate: This is an excellent procedure if you have thick surface veins that appear to bulge. If you have had endovenous laser therapy, ambulatory phlebectomy is a good follow-up treatment to remove your bulging surface veins.

How Often: Once.
Cost: $750.

MOST COMMONLY ASKED QUESTIONS

Question: Will all of my superficial leg vein problems be treated in a single session?

Answer: If you are having sclerotherapy, which is considered to be the most effective way to treat unsightly superficial leg veins, you may have to undergo several treatments, depending on the number of problem veins you have. Typically, the physician will inject no more that fifteen veins on each leg per session.

Question: I understand sclerotherapy requires multiple injections. Will this hurt?

Answer: The needles used to inject the solution into the tiny spider veins on the legs are very fine. Because they are also being injected just under the skin, the treatment is rarely painful. However, towards the end of a session, you may begin to experience some discomfort.

Chapter 8

Face, Brow, and Eye Lifts

As we age, not only do we have to deal with lines, wrinkles, broken blood vessels, and brown spots, but we also have to cope with sagging, loose skin. For the most part, we have gravity to thank, and while this force of nature may keep our feet planted firmly on the ground, it is also why every other part of our body tends to head south over time. It's no secret that astronauts look years younger in space. Without gravity to weigh them down, it's as if years were literally lifted off their faces. Once back on planet Earth, however, they have to deal with the hanging jowls, turkey necks, bags under the eyes, and droopy foreheads just like the rest of us.

Although you can erase some of the outward signs of aging with nonsurgical procedures such as lasers, fillers, and injectables, none of these techniques can compare to surgical procedures when it comes to lifting and tightening the skin. Unlike the subtle improvements that Thermage and Botox can provide, surgery such as a face, brow, or eyelid lift will provide an immediate and long-lasting transformation that will be noticeable and dramatic. While lifts won't change the texture of your skin or remove fine lines and wrinkles around the lips and eyes, they will reduce the amount of sagging skin. By decreasing the amount of loose skin and fat on the neck, jaw line, brow, or eyelid, lifts will result in a firmer and younger-looking face.

Even in this day and age, there are people performing facelifts and other such procedures who have no surgical training (see Chapter 15, "Choosing a Qualified Specialist"). So be warned. In your consultation, ask for proof of your physician's qualifications and experience. This is your face—and potentially your life—that you are trusting to an individual, who may be totally incompetent when it comes to performing surgery of this nature. Make certain beyond a doubt that he or she is qualified to perform such an operation.

FACELIFT (RHYTIDECTOMY)

Background: The first recorded facelift (rhytidectomy) was performed in 1901 by a Dr. Hollander. A rather crude predecessor to today's surgery, this turn-of-the-last-century technique basically involved cutting away the excess skin in front of the patient's ears. Then in 1910, another physician by the name of Lexer developed a procedure that cut the skin, lifted it away from the underlying tissue (called a skin flap), and then pulled it back. Over the course of the next sixty years, this face-lifting technique remained relatively unchanged except for a few minor improvements that helped to conceal the scars. It wasn't until 1974 that Dr. Skoog came up with the basic system that is used today, in which the deeper layers of muscle (called the submuscular aponeurotic system—SMAS) that lay below the skin are also pulled up. By lifting this layer of muscle, which has lost its bulk, removing excess skin and re-draping it, the procedure should result in a natural-looking appearance that can take up to ten years off your face.

Patients have a few options when deciding to proceed with a facelift. It can be performed in the traditional open

Chapter 8| Face, Brow, and Eye Lifts

method described below or by endoscopic surgery, which allows the surgeon to operate through a narrow tube called a cannula, while viewing the operation through a camera. Because they are less invasive, leave fewer scars, and result in a shorter healing period, endoscopic facelifts are popular for those who have mild to moderate sagging of the skin. You can also choose to have what is known as a mini-facelift, which only treats the face, as opposed to a full facelift that treats the face and the neck. People often opt to combine a facelift with other procedures, such as eyelid surgery, a brow lift, fillers, peels, or laser resurfacing. All of these options should be discussed with your surgeon during your consultation.

Technique: Before deciding on this operation, you must be candid with your surgeon about your health history. If you have heart disease, high blood pressure, disorders that inhibit the blood from clotting, and any wound healing problems associated with the likes of diabetes, lupus, or HIV, you will be at a much higher risk for complications during the operation. Smokers should quit for at least six weeks before and after the operation, since serious complications related to smoking can occur after the operation, such as improper healing due to blood vessel constriction, infection, and skin sloughing. People under high risk will not necessarily be deterred from having a facelift, but they must accept these dangers (see the full list of complications on page 113 and 114). If the surgeon agrees to the operation, he or she will most likely handle the procedure more conservatively. Aspirin or other acetylsalicylic acid products should not be taken for two weeks prior to the operation, since the medication thins the blood and can cause increased bleeding and bruising.

A facelift is most often conducted in a hospital, but may also be done in a clinic setting. It is usually performed using either a local anaesthetic with an intravenous sedation or a general anaesthetic. If you are having a traditional facelift, a continuous incision will be made around the ear before the skin is lifted. Another incision will be made under the chin if the neck is to be corrected, and if there are thick bands in the neck they may have to be tied or folded together. The muscle layer under the skin of the face and neck is then tightened and, at this time, fat may be extracted by surgery or by liposuction (see Chapter 10, "Body Contouring"). The skin is then pulled over the face and re-draped, and any excess skin is cut away. Different surgeons will have varying techniques, which may even vary from patient to patient. While some surgeons may choose to make an incision in front of the hairline, others may cut in or behind the hair. It is recommended that you talk to your surgeon beforehand about his or her individual method and what your specific needs may be (see figure below).

If an endoscopic facelift is performed, minimal points of access will be made to accommodate the tube that allows the lighted camera and surgical instruments to pass under

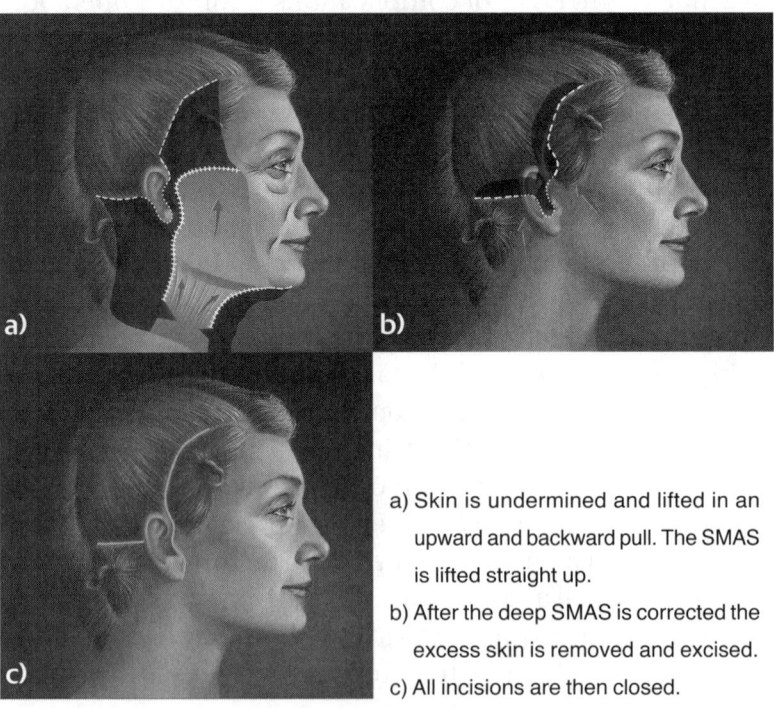

a) Skin is undermined and lifted in an upward and backward pull. The SMAS is lifted straight up.
b) After the deep SMAS is corrected the excess skin is removed and excised.
c) All incisions are then closed.

Chapter 8| Face, Brow, and Eye Lifts

the skin. In this procedure, the surgeon will lift everything above the bone as a single unit. Skin layering may also be combined with the endoscopic technique.

Although some facelifts are performed on an outpatient basis, meaning you can go home the same day after the operation, many hospitals and clinics will keep you in for twenty-four hours. A tube, which will drain any fluids that may collect under the skin, is often inserted at the hairline on the back of the neck and will usually remain in for twenty-four to forty-eight hours. The entire procedure should take anywhere between two to four hours, depending on the amount of work you are having done.

Downtime: Two to four weeks. After a week, you will be able to go out of the house, but because the bruising and swelling will still be very apparent, you will most likely want to wear some type of concealing coverage such as a hat, sunglasses, and scarf. After two weeks, you may return to work wearing makeup to cover any discoloration. If you don't want anyone to know that you've had a facelift, then you should plan to book a month away from your normal activities. Endoscopic facelifts will heal faster than a traditional facelift, but will still have significant bruising and swelling.

Complications: If you have the procedure under a general anaesthesia, there will be the usual associated risks, especially during a longer surgery, such as deep leg clots that can break off and go to the lungs. There is also the danger of fluid collecting (such as hematomas) under the skin, which may compromise wound healing.

Expect medium to mild pain after the facelift, which should subside within twenty-four hours. There will also be swelling and bruising of the entire face that may last for up to two weeks. There is also a low risk of infection and skin slough around the incisions, especially higher if you are a smoker and haven't quit before and/or after the operation. This sloughing occurs when the skin has lost its blood supply due to vessels that have constricted. The result of a lack of blood will cause the skin to die and turn a crusty black. When the scab-like formation eventually falls off, it will reveal an open wound in the skin. If the hole is small, it may heal on its own, but if it is large, a second surgery, which can even require a skin graft, may have to take place. Asymmetry of the face is also possible.

There is also a less than 1 percent risk that the sensory (feeling nerves) or motor (muscle nerves) nerves might be damaged during the operation. If the sensory nerve is affected, you might get some numbness in the area, but it should subside in time. The most common visual sign that a motor nerve has been damaged is a droopy lower lip, which in 98 percent of all cases, disappears after a few weeks to months.

Irregularities and rippling, or little lumps and bumps under the skin, may occur and they can be dealt with by gently massaging the affected area. You may also have to change your hairstyle to conceal any scars, which may initially appear white or red, or thick. Loss of hair near the scars may also occur.

A more common complication that may happen in the weeks following a facelift is mild and temporary depression. Caused by unrealistic expectations, anxiety, or frustration with the healing process, the despondency usually disappears once the visual and full results of the facelift are obvious, which can take from weeks to months to a year.

Post-treatment: Rest with the head elevated is recommended for the first couple of days at home. If you have had your neck done, be careful not to bend it by laying on a pillow, since it can impede the blood supply of the neck skin. Use ice to counteract the swelling, and a medication such as Tylenol 3, which will be prescribed by your physician, to control the pain. Once the drainage tube is out, you may shower and wash your hair with a mild shampoo, but the use of a blow dryer or any heat near your face is not recommended for at least two weeks. Nor is the use of makeup advised, especially on the incisions, for that same period of time. Some of the sutures will be removed on the third day after the operation, and the rest will come out on the fifth day. Even though the sutures will have been long removed, you should not colour your hair for at least a month. Although you may resume mild exercise such as walking within a few days, no strenuous physical exertion should take place until four to six weeks after the operation.

Results: A facelift that has been done properly should smooth, lift, and tighten any loose skin and underlying tissues on your face and neck. While it will not remove fine lines and wrinkles around your eyes and mouth, other larger wrinkles will appear diminished. Overall, a facelift has the capability of eradicating approximately ten years from your face, and the effects should last for about ten years.

If a facelift has been performed improperly resulting in a "too tight" look, surgeons can improve on it but can't totally reverse the tautness, since new skin cannot be added. However, if you go to a qualified, experienced surgeon, you should get a facelift that will look good for ten years as opposed to one that will take ten years to look good.

Ideal Candidate: If you have sagging jowls, loose skin on the neck, and/or bands of thick muscle lines, you can definitely benefit from a traditional facelift. To see if this operation is for you, lie down and look up at a mirror. Those are the results you can expect with a facelift.

How Often: Once. Although many facelifts can be performed on an individual, only a single operation should be required to achieve results that will last for approximately ten years.

Cost: $13,500–$15,000.

FOREHEAD (BROW LIFT)

Background: Performed in 1919 by Dr. Passot, the first recorded brow lift involved making an incision in the hairline and pulling the skin back to remove the laxity around the outer part of the eyebrow, called the lateral brow. Then in 1930, other physicians began to experiment with incising in the middle of the forehead to correct the overall droopiness of the brow. Soon after, the method that was still popular until the late 1990s was developed, whereby an incision was made within the hairline that ran straight across the top of the head from ear to ear. After being lifted, any loose skin was excised. In more recent years, however, the endoscopic brow lift was universalized, and in most cases has replaced the conventional brow lift surgery. Less invasive, an endoscopic brow lift results in fewer scars, complications, and a quick recovery period.

Often performed in combination with a facelift and eyelid surgery, the brow lift will improve and soften lines in the forehead that often make us look angry or tired. It will also reposition the eyebrows slightly higher on the face. Ideally, women's eyebrows should sit at the bony edge above the eye or higher, while men's brows should sit at the edge or lower. There should be a nice arch in the brow, with the middle (medial) brow being slightly lower than the lateral brow. In other words, the eyebrows should tilt up and out. A properly performed brow lift will accomplish this and will also improve the look of the upper eyelids. The overall effect will be a more youthful, rested, and relaxed appearance.

Technique: Seven to twelve days before your scheduled surgery, you will often receive a Botox injection to relax the forehead muscles. The brow lift will be performed under a general anaesthetic in a hospital or at a clinic, and often at the same time as a facelift. The surgeon will either execute the traditional operation, as outlined above, or use an endoscope, making three to five small incisions. During the operation, a drainage tube may be been inserted in the skin to collect any fluids, and will remain there for twenty-four hours. If you are being treated on an outpatient basis, you will be able to go home the same day after the operation. However, some hospitals and clinics will keep you in overnight. The procedure should take approximately one to two hours to

Chapter 8| **Face, Brow, and Eye Lifts** 117

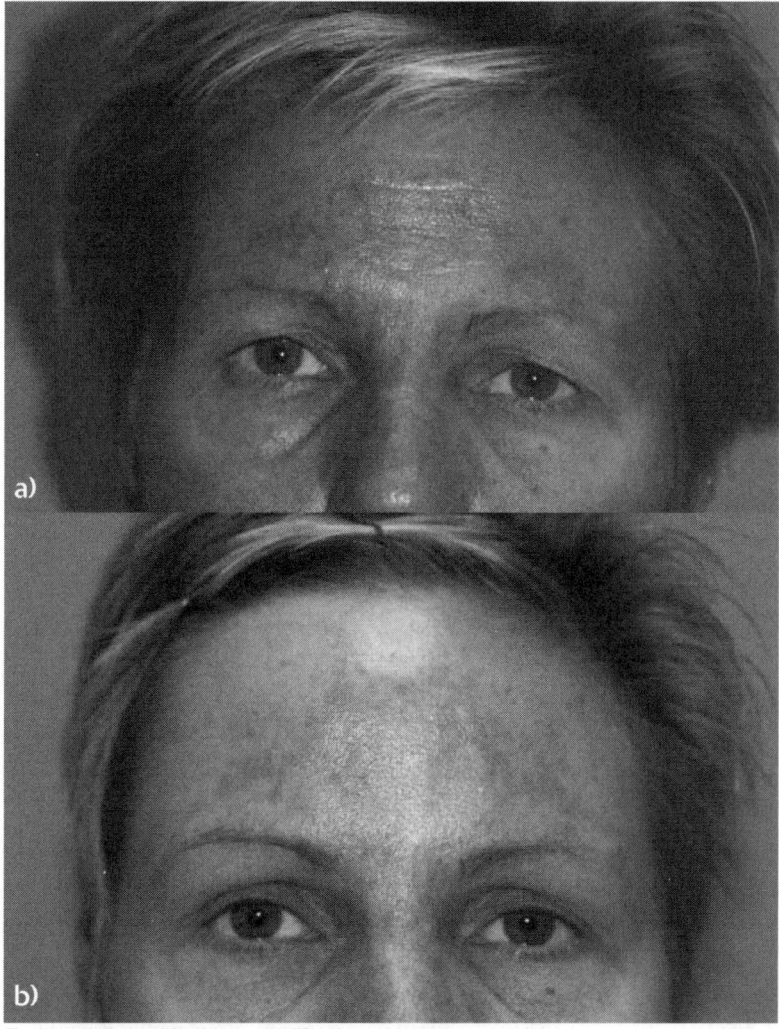

Endoscopic brow lift with eyelid lift. a) pre b) post

perform, but the duration will depend on the type of surgery and the amount of work being done.

Downtime: If you have had a traditional brow lift, expect to be away from your normal routine for at least seven to ten days. An endoscopic brow lift will usually only require four to seven days of downtime.

Complications: You may have a moderate to severe headache for forty-eight hours after the operation, and there may also be pain around the incised areas. The brow will appear shiny, swollen, and tight for the first two weeks, and the skin surrounding both of your eyes may be bruised. Although occurring in less than 1 percent of patients, infection, hematomas, numbness, and a droopy brow are associated risks with a brow lift. All the aforementioned complications are most often transient, meaning that if they occur, they will usually improve with time. Noticeable white, or red, thick, raised scars may also be apparent, and permanent hair loss around the scar areas may occur.

Post-treatment: A medication such as Tylenol 3 may be prescribed for the headache and pain around the incisions. The head should be elevated during rest periods for as long as the swelling is presant.

Results: There will be an improvement in the upper eyelids and the positioning of the eyebrows. The forehead will appear smoother and the vertical lines between the brows, known as the glabella, will soften.

Ideal Candidate: If your brows seem to be sitting lower or too close to the eyes you are probably a good candidate for a brow lift. You would also benefit from this surgery if you have deep vertical lines in the glabella or transverse lines across the forehead. To pre-determine if a brow lift would improve your appearance, pull your eyebrows up. If you don't look shocked or surprised, and see an improvement in your upper eyelids, you will probably like the results of this surgery.

How Often: Usually once (depends on how you age).

Cost: $6,500–$7,500.

EYELID LIFT (BLEPHAROPLASTY)

Background: Because the skin loses its elasticity as we grow older, and the excess skin and fat above and below the eye become more pronounced and baggy, it is most often this area of our face that seems to age the fastest. Eyelid lift surgery, called a blepharoplasty, is the most effective way to correct this problem. One of the most common of all cosmetic surgical procedures, there is evidence

Chapter 8| Face, Brow, and Eye Lifts 119

that eyelid surgery to correct droopy eyelids was being performed in Arabia as far back as 980. However, it wasn't until 1844 that the first cosmetic eyelid surgery was recorded.

Often performed with a face or a brow lift, an eyelid lift can be done on either the upper eyelid, if there is too much skin between the brow and the eye, or the lower eyelid to correct puffy or baggy eyes. However, there are several conditions that it won't improve, including dark circles, an uneven opening of the eye, disorders

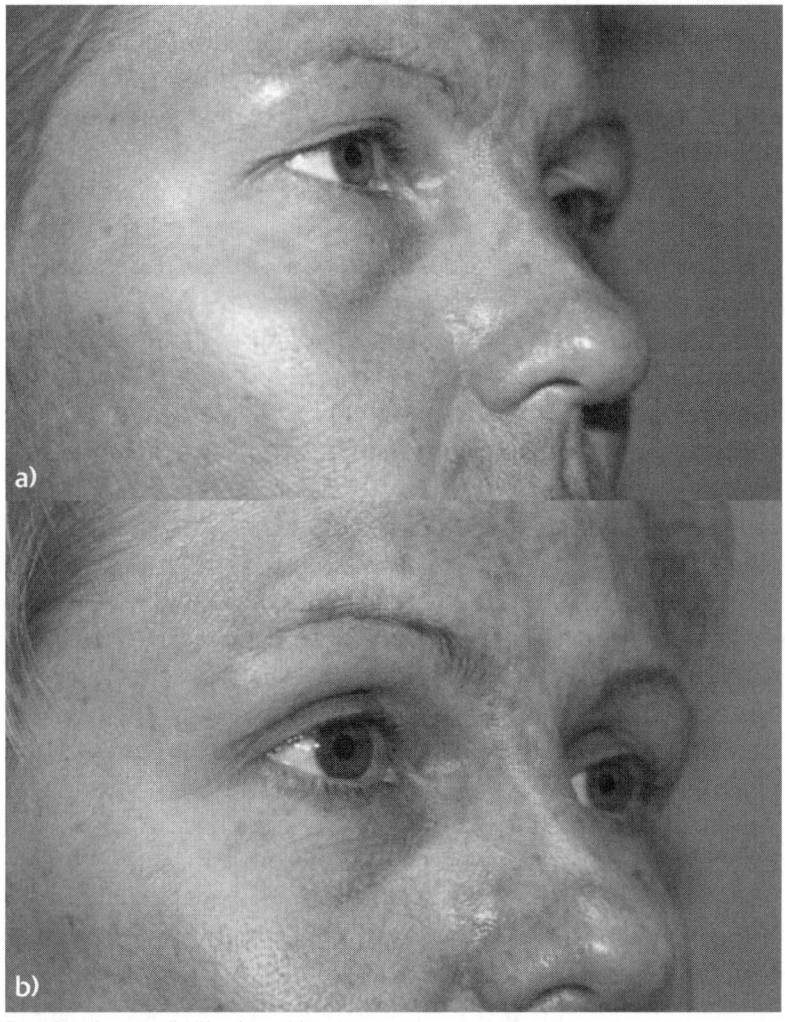

Results of an eyelid lift. a) pre b) post

that causes dry eyes, or bulging eyes due to thyroid disease. In fact, if a blepharoplasty was performed in an attempt to correct bulging eyes, it will most likely worsen the problem.

Anyone with bleeding problems, diabetes, high blood pressure, glaucoma or other serious vision problems may be at higher risk during this operation (see complications below), so it is very important to discuss your health history with your surgeon.

Technique: Both upper and lower eyelid surgery are performed under a local anaesthetic and possibly with intravenous sedation if needed. If the upper eyelid is being done, an incision will be made along the crease line and above to remove the required amount of excess skin. A tiny strip of exposed muscle may then be removed in order to create a deeper eye crease. After this has been completed, any excess fat under the muscle will also be removed from the two exposed fat pads. Sutures will be used to close the incisions.

The lower eyelid may be corrected by using either the external technique, in which an incision is made just below the eyelashes to remove excess skin, muscle, and fat, or the transconjunctival technique, which eliminates only the fatty pockets. If the latter of the two operations is being performed, the incision will be made on the inside of the eyelid, leaving no visible scars. Whether you are having the upper and/or lower eyelid surgery, it will usually take no longer than an hour, and you will not require an overnight stay at the hospital or clinic.

Downtime: One to two weeks.

Complications: There may be bruising and swelling around the eyes, but both of these after-effects will disappear within two weeks. If you are healthy and a nonsmoker, or have quit smoking for six weeks prior to and six weeks after the operation, severe complications are rare during and after an eyelid lift. However, there is a slight risk of bleeding that can incite a blood clot to form within the eye socket. This bleeding behind the eye and subsequent pressure on the eye and nerves can cause changes in

Chapter 8| Face, Brow, and Eye Lifts

vision or even blindness but is very rare. Infection, irritation of the cornea, scarring, a turning inward or outward of the eyelashes, numbness, a lack of symmetry between the two eyes, and loss of movement of the eyelid are also possible uncommon risks. If an external lower eye lift was performed, there is a chance that the resulting scar may cause the eyelid to be pulled downward. Called scleral show, the lower whites of the eye will be exposed in an unnatural manner. Gentle massage that pushes the lower eyelid up can usually correct this problem if mild, however, in more severe cases, another surgery may have to be performed.

Post-treatment: You will be given an ice pack by the doctor to counteract the swelling, and it is recommended that you continue to apply cold or ice packs until the swelling has subsided. Sleep and rest with the head elevated for at least a couple of days. Any pain should be minimal to moderate, but you can take medication such as Tylenol 3 if needed. Although the stitches will be removed within three to five days, contact lenses are not to be worn for one to two weeks.

Results: Droopiness and puffiness between the brow and the eye will have disappeared along with the excess skin and fat if an upper eyelid surgery was performed. Any puffiness and sagging below the eye should also be removed with lower eyelid surgery.

Ideal Candidate: If you have loose, baggy or puffy skin above or below the eyes, you are a good candidate for an eyelid lift.

How Often: Once to achieve results that can last for up to ten years.

Cost: $4,000–$5,000 for upper and lower eyelids; $2,000–$3,000 for either upper or lower eyelids.

MOST COMMONLY ASKED QUESTIONS

Question: I've had techniques performed such as Thermage, Featherlift, and fillers. Can I have a facelift after having these other procedures done?

Answer: Yes. Furthermore, you can even have these treatments

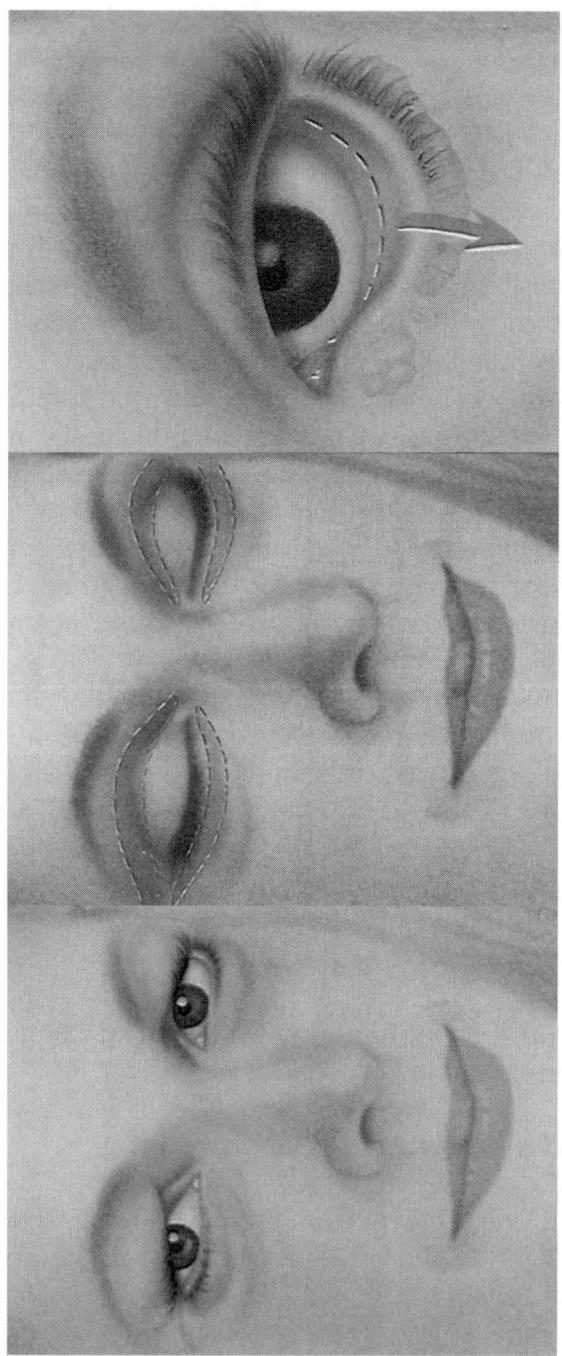

a) Excess loose skin and bulging of the fat around the eyes occur with aging.

b) For eyelid lifts the incisions are placed in the natural creases of the eyelids. Through these incisions loose skin and excess fat can be removed.

c) In transconjunctival blepharoplasty an incision is made on the inside of the eyelid and the fatty pockets are corrected. There is no external scar but there is also no removal of skin.

Chapter 8| Face, Brow, and Eye Lifts

done after a facelift in order to maintain the results and prolong the need for repeat surgery.

Question: I'm a smoker and I've heard that facelifts are unsafe for someone who smokes. Is this true?

Answer: Smoking can cause the small blood vessels to go into spasm, and when the skin is lifted during the surgery, the skin at the incision edge may not have enough blood supply to survive, resulting in the possibility of large areas of skin loss. Infection rates are also higher in smokers. Therefore, ideally you should stop smoking for at least six weeks prior to the surgery and for at least six weeks afterwards.

Question: I have heard that a brow lift will make you look surprised. Is this true?

Answer: Brow lifts are used to reposition the brow in relationship to the upper end of the orbital bone. Brows should be placed in a natural position and not excessively pulled, as the result will be an abnormality to the face.

Question: I cannot open my eyes fully. Can this be corrected with an eyelid lift?

Answer: Eyelid surgery will not treat the decreased ability to open the eyelid (called ptosis). This condition must be corrected by treating the underlying muscles or the medical cause. If surgical correction is needed it can be done in combination with an eyelid lift if it is required.

Question: I'm not sure if I need a brow lift or an eyelid lift. How can I determine this?

Answer: Your surgeon will look at your eyebrow position while it is at rest (as you relax your face and brow). When the brow is in this neutral position, then the surgeon can determine if the brow is sitting in a good place and whether there is excess upper eyelid skin. If you have a droopy forehead often the muscles in your brow are very active in an attempt to hold the forehead and loose eyelid skin away from your eyes. When the excess loose eyelid skin is removed without correcting the droopy brow the muscles of the forehead often relax (because there is less skin overhanging the eyes) and the brow droop actually appears worse than before surgery.

Question: Can I have an eyelid lift if I've had laser vision correction?

Answer: Yes. After conferring with the specialist who performed the laser vision correction, to ensure there are no outstanding concerns, an eyelid lift can be performed eight to twelve weeks afterwards.

Chapter 9

Facial
Contouring

While the eyes may be the windows to the soul, the size and shape of our nose, chin, and ears make a huge impact on how we are perceived by others. High cheekbones denote an air of sophistication and glamour, while a broad jaw line represents commanding strength. The owner of a tiny, turned-up nose is deemed to be fun-loving, yet if the same person had a long, straight nose, he or she may be considered haughty or regal in their bearing. People with large, floppy ears are sometimes presumed to be of less intelligence, and no matter how confident, strong-willed, or determined a person is, if they have a receding chin, they are often presumed to be weak.

In reality, facial features have nothing to do with our personalities and almost always are determined by genetics, including racial background. Nevertheless, if we are treated in a certain manner over the course of many years because others perceive us to be that way, it may eventually become a self-fulfilling prophecy. If you're unhappy about a certain part of your face, it can affect the way you present yourself to the world.

Plastic surgeons have long been the experts in correcting certain facial features that may be bothering us, and have adopted a generally standardized approach. The majority of them maintain that in order for the face to be aesthetically pleasing, each feature should be in balance with one another. While looking at your face in profile, the surgeon will visually divide it into the following three segments:

- *Upper face:* Forehead, brow, upper eyelids
- *Mid-level face:* Lower eyelids, cheeks, nose, ears
- *Lower face:* Mouth, chin, jaw, neck

After carefully evaluating the size, shape and structure of each of your facial features, he or she can then determine if an area is out of balance or in disharmony with the rest of the face. For example, you may be unhappy with the size of your nose, believing it to be too big. However, after analysis, the surgeon may deem that your chin is actually too small in comparison to the rest of the facial features. By reconstructing the chin's shape and size, the nose that you thought to be too prominent will fall into balance with the rest of your face.

Most facial contouring involves reshaping either the cheeks, nose, ears, or chin, and the overall medical term for all of these procedures is profiloplasty. Implants or fat injections (see Chapter 6, "Wrinkles") can be used to heighten the cheekbone area, and the chin can be augmented by either implants or bone restructuring, which is called a sliding genioplasty. Ears are usually surgically corrected through otoplasty, which reshapes the cartilage. Noses are refigured in a variety of ways, called rhinoplasty. Noses can either be enlarged by using implants or adding cartilage, or decreased in size by surgically reconstructing the base.

Whatever your concern, the first step in correcting the problem is to consult with a surgeon who is qualified and experienced in facial surgery. He or she will evaluate your facial profile and discuss feasible options. Often, more than one procedure may be necessary and can usually be done at the same time. As with any surgery, there are several complications that can arise during or after an operation, so discussing your health history with your doctor prior to making any decisions is of the utmost importance.

CHEEK (MALAR) AUGMENTATION

Background: Cheek augmentation, which raises the cheekbone and give it a forward projection, can also improve the look of the lower eyelid area. This procedure can be done by taking fat from your own body (called an autogenous technique), and injecting it into the cheek area, or by implanting a foreign substance (called an alloplastic technique), such as solid silicone next to the bone. The operation is often performed in conjunction with a rhinoplasty and/or a facelift. If the autogenous technique is used, the injections will be given after liposuction (see Chapter 10, "Body Contouring").

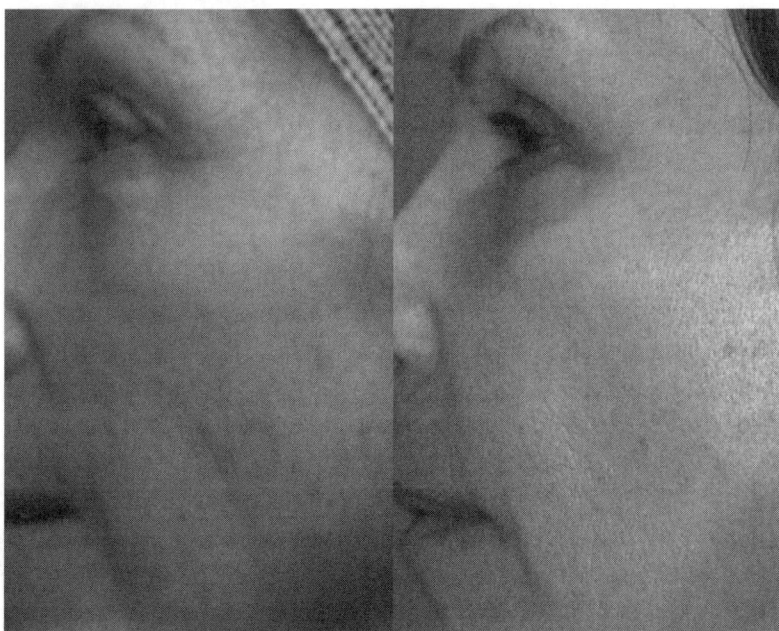

Pre and post cheek silicone implants.

Using the body's own fat to build up the area is the most versatile method of augmentation because it is a relatively easy procedure for the surgeon to perform. And unless the person is very thin, the fat supply is usually plentiful enough for the surgeon to obtain the amount they will require for the augmentation. Sometimes bone will also be used to build up the cheek area, but this is usually reserved for when there has been extensive trauma to the face as opposed to straightforward cosmetic enhancements. However, the problem in using autogenous tissue of any kind, whether it be fat, bone, muscle, cartilage, or skin, is that the surgeon has to borrow it from a donor site. This means that instead of having a single wound and scar to deal with, there will be two areas that will have to heal. In the case of a cheek augmentation for cosmetic purposes, the fat is usually taken through liposuction from the hips, stomach, or thighs and then injected into the face. Although the injections will have relatively few complications, there are risks associated with liposuction. Furthermore, there can be up to a 50 percent loss of the fat after it has been injected into the cheek area, which will most likely result in a second procedure a year later.

Alloplastic surgery in the form of cheek (malar) implants is becoming an increasingly popular way to enlarge and heighten the area. Considered to be a fairly uncomplicated procedure, it is most often done from inside of the mouth, which leaves no visible scar. Surgeons used such foreign materials as gold and bone to implant under the skin at the turn of the last century, but modern medicine now incorporates a wide range of materials, such as various forms of carbon-based polymers, metals such as titanium, and ceramics. However, the most common type of implant currently used in augmentation procedures are noncarbon-based polymers in the form of silicone, or silastic. Although there has been much publicity regarding the issue of silicone implants, especially when used for breast augmentation, (see Chapter 12, "Breast Enhancements"), there is actually no solid evidence linking silicone to systemic medical conditions. In fact, there are many advantages in using this type of implant since the substance is highly resistant to degradation and presents no known toxicity or allergic reactions. As with any alloplastic procedure, however, there is always the danger of infection and the chance that the implant may be pushed out by the body (called extrusion), which happens when the body rejects the foreign substance.

An interesting side note is that many people believe the term "plastic surgeon" is used because these surgeons use plastics. But in reality, the word "plastic" comes from the Greek word *plastikos*, which means to mould or to sculpt. During World War I, surgeons attempted to repair and reconstruct the bodies and faces of soldiers who suffered devastating deformities. Because they were re-moulding or re-shaping their patients, these surgeons became known as plastic surgeons.

Technique: If fat injections are to be used, liposuction will be conducted first. Performed under a local anaesthetic, fat is taken from your own body and then implanted into your cheek area with multiple injections. If a silicone implant is being used, the procedure will most likely be performed through an incision in the mouth. This is the preferred method because it will not leave a visable scar. If the incision is made on the outside of the face it is usually placed under the lower eyelashes. Also performed under a local anesthetic and taking about 20 minutes to execute on each cheek, the surgeon will make an incision on the gums between the upper lip and teeth. The tissue above the bone will then be lifted, and a pocket will be made for the implant, which will then be inserted. The pocket will be closed with sutures.

Downtime: Seven days away from your normal routine will be required for either fat injections or silicone implants.

Complications: There will be the risks associated with liposuction if fat injections are used (see Chapter 10). With both types of procedures, swelling, bruising, and some discomfort will occur for about a week. If a foreign implant has been inserted, there will also be the risk of infection; possible malposition of the implant, which may require a second surgery to correct; bleeding at the surgical site; extrusion of the implant, temporary nerve injury in the form of loss of feeling or muscle movement, and long-term bone erosion, which can occur from the effects of a solid foreign object sitting against the bone.

Post-treatment: Mild pain medication may be taken for the discomfort that is associated with either procedure. The treated area should remain as relatively still as possible for seven days, meaning no rubbing or exaggerated facial expressions. If an incision was made in the mouth, you should rinse with salt water after every meal, eat only soft foods, and do not chew gum for about a week.

Results: Cheek implants can lift the whole face, and may also improve the lower eyelid area and the laugh lines and even occasionally the jowls.

Ideal Candidate: If your cheeks are weak or lower than you would like, then you would be a good candidate for cheek augmentation.

How Often: Fat injections will require a second procedure after a year, while silicone implants will only need to be done once unless there is a complication, which requires a second operation.

Cost: $4,500–$5,500 (for both implants and injections, which may include the cost of liposuction).

CHIN RESHAPING (MENTOPLASTY)

Background: The preferred ways to augment or reshape the chin are either by inserting a solid silicone implant next to the bone, or by using a procedure called a sliding genioplasty, which involves cutting the bone and moving it forward to correct a receding chin or by moving it backward to diminish a large chin. If the bite of the teeth is not aligned properly, however, corrective jaw (orthognathic) or orthodontic surgery may be required before chin reshaping can be considered. In addition, there may be problems with the jaw as opposed to the chin, and this will

Chapter 9| Facial Contouring

need to be addressed in the form of a jaw enhancement, where the entire lower jaw, chin, and teeth are moved forward. Chin reshaping is often combined with a rhinoplasty.

Technique: If an implant is being used, the operation will be performed under a local anaesthetic and will take approximately forty-five minutes. A small incision will be made under the chin or inside the mouth on the gumline between the lower lip and the teeth. A pocket will then be created in which the implant is inserted. Once the implant is in place, the incision will be closed with sutures. Using an incision under the chin may reduce the risk of infection that can occur inside the mouth, but it will leave a small, visible scar under the chin.

The sliding genioplasty is used when it is necessary to move the chin either forward or backward. This procedure is performed with either a general anaesthetic or a local anaesthetic with an intravenous sedation and takes up to two hours. The surgeon

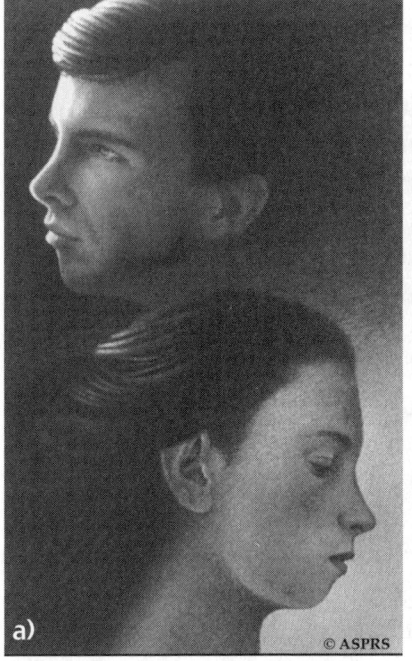
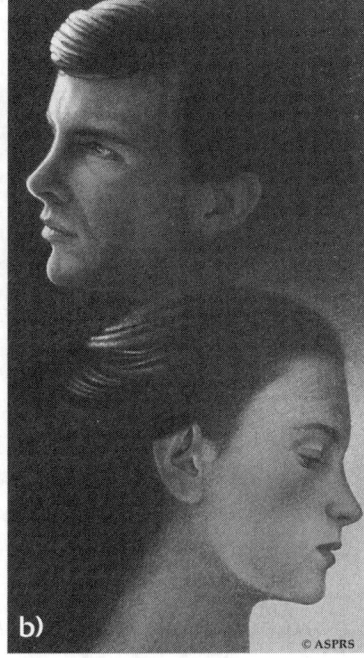

a) A weak chin can cause significant imbalance in patients facial profile.

b) Chin implants can dramatically improve facial balance with minimal downtime.

will usually operate from the inside of your mouth (although the procedure can also be performed from under the chin), and use your own bone tissue to adjust the chin. The surgeon cuts the bone along the edge of the lower teeth to release the area from the rest of the jawbone. At this stage the surgeon will either cut the bone to shorten the chin or move it forward about ½ to 1 centimetre to lengthen the chin. It may also be adjusted up or down, depending on the desired reshaping. When the operation is near completion, the new bone adjustment will be secured in place by screws or plates, and the incision will be closed.

Downtime: Seven to ten days will be required before you resume normal activities. Swelling may last longer.

Complications: If you have had a chin implant, expect mild to moderate discomfort and swelling for seven days. Risks associated with a chin implant can include infection; bleeding at the site; malpositioning of the implant, which may have to be corrected with a second surgery; a temporary numbness or loss of movement in the area due to nerve damage; and long-term bone erosion.

If you have had your chin adjusted with a sliding genioplasty, expect some discomfort that can last for up to two weeks. The most common complication of this operation is temporary numbness in the area. A lesser risk would be infection, and bone loss caused by the loss of blood supply when the bone was separated from the rest of the jaw.

Post-treatment: With either operation, rinse the mouth with salt water for several days afterwards, and a soft diet is recommended. Do not chew gum and avoid any unnecessary movement of the area for at least a week. Medication such as Tylenol 3 can be taken for any pain.

Results: When a chin implant is inserted, a receding or weak chin will have more prominence. If the chin has been adjusted through a sliding genioplasty, a long chin will be shortened or a small chin will be lengthened. The tip of the chin can also be tilted upwards to shorten the face, or downwards to lengthen it.

Ideal Candidate: If you have any concerns regarding the size or shape of your chin, you may want to consider either operation.
How Often: Once for augmentation or reshaping, unless there is a complication, which requires a second operation.
Cost: $2,500–$3,500 for a chin implant; $3,500–$6,000 for a sliding genioplasty.

NOSE RESHAPING (RHINOPLASTY)

Background: Reconstructive surgery on the nose was first described in India and Egypt as far back as 600 B.C. However, it wasn't until 1887 that a true cosmetic nose correction was performed in New York City by a Dr. Roe. Although this surgery is one of the most common aesthetic procedures being done, it is considered to be technically difficult because it is performed with limited visibility. Furthermore, because the surgeon is altering the architecture of the nose, or reconstructing the bone and cartilage without cutting any skin, it takes time to see the final results. The skin may tighten or contract, and although there will be some immediate improvement in the overall shape of the nose, the results of how the skin will react may not be seen for up to a year after the operation.

Often combined with a septoplasty, which repairs a deviated septum, or a chin augmentation to improve facial balance, one of the main concerns involving a rhinoplasty is the unrealistic expectations of the patient. If you are looking for an exact replica of the nose of a movie star or model, you will most likely be disappointed with the results. Although your nose can be made smaller or larger, it is nearly impossible for the surgeon to recreate someone else's nose. Repeated rhinoplastys due to patient dissatisfaction or a surgeon attempting to achieve a patient's unrealistic desires can result in what physicians call "the over-operated nose." Indeed, severe deformities can take place when several nose operations are performed, so it is vital that you see a surgeon who is very experienced in rhinoplasty.

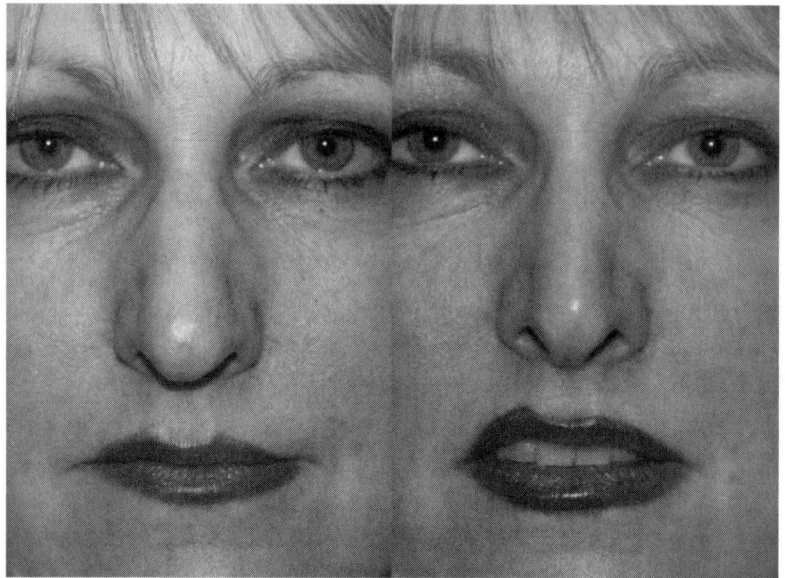
Pre and post rhinoplasty

Technique: Aspirin and other medications containing acetylsalicylic acid should not be taken for seven days before the procedure. Depending on the complexity of the operation, it can take up to two hours to perform and you will be given either a general anaesthetic or a local anaesthetic with an intravenous sedation. The operation will either be performed in what is called a closed rhinoplasty, in which two incisions are made on the inside of the nose, or an open rhinoplasty, which consists of the two internal incisions plus another incision across the base of the nose. The skin of the entire nose will then be flipped up so the base architecture of the nose is exposed. At this stage, the reconstruction is achieved by removing or remoulding bone and cartilage. Often, the bone of the nose is cut and repositioned during the procedure. Once this reconstruction has been completed, the skin will be put back in place and the incisions will be closed with sutures. The nose will then be packed with gauze and a cast, splint, or tape may also be applied.
Downtime: One to two weeks.

Chapter 9| **Facial Contouring** 135

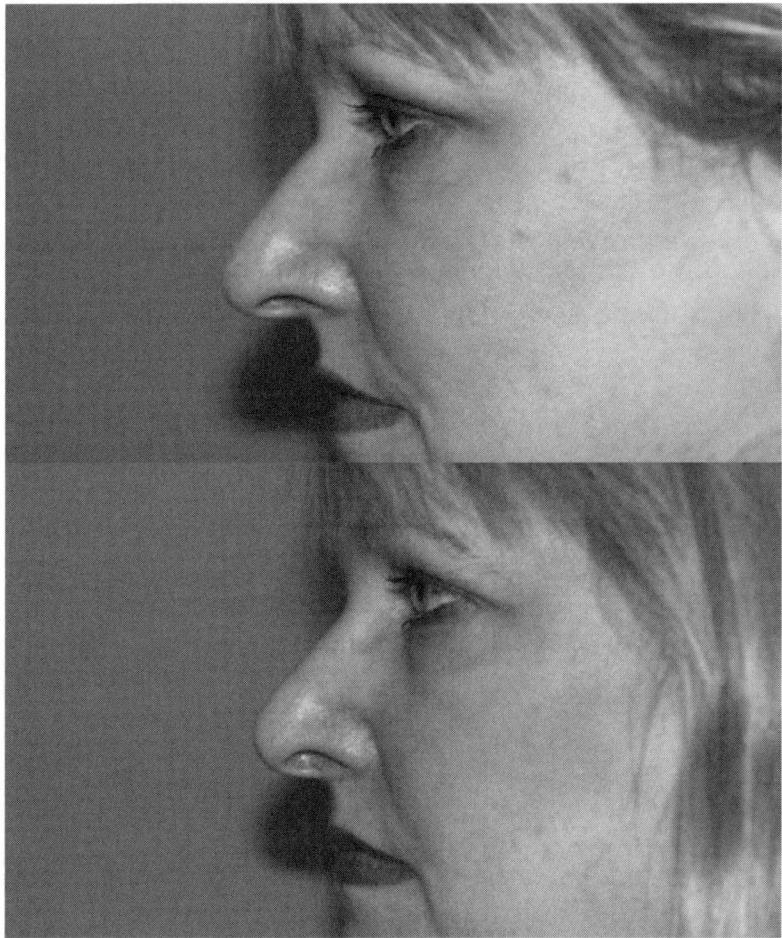

Pre and post rhinoplasty.

Complications: There will be swelling and bruising around the nose and eye area, which will generally subside after two weeks. However, in some cases, swelling can persist for up to a year. The risk associated with a rhinoplasty is bleeding. Although rare, infection may also occur. In highly sensitive people, allergic reactions to the tape and other minor skin complications may occur. Spider veins are another common occurrence after a rhinoplasty, as are nasal obstructions, which are mostly seen immediately following the operation and tend to clear up on their own after a couple of weeks. There also may be a temporary loss of smell, which can last from six to eighteen months, and in a few rare cases, it may be permanent. The skin over the nose may initially seem loose, especially in patients over the age of fifty. It will tighten in time and results will not fully be seen for twelve months after the surgery.

Post-treatment: Rest with the head elevated is recommended for the first day after the procedure. Medication such as Tylenol 3 may be taken for any discomfort. The packing will be removed within two to three days, but the cast or splint will remain on the nose for seven to ten days.

Results: After a rhinoplasty, the nose will either be smaller, larger, or reshaped to be more aesthetically pleasing. The skin response to the new nose will not be complete until 1 year postoperatively.

Ideal Candidate: If you believe your nose is out of balance with the rest of your face, this procedure may be of benefit to you.

How Often: Rate of requiring further surgical enhancement is 15 percent at one year.

Cost: $5,500–$6,500.

EAR SURGERY
Split Earlobes

Background: There are several operations that can be performed on the ears to resolve congenital problems, but there are only two common surgeries that are currently being conducted for cosmetic enhancement. The first is in the repairing of earlobes that have been split or near-split from the constant wearing of heavy pierced earrings. This type of split may also be caused from an earring accidentally being ripped from the earlobe. The surgery may also be performed on earlobes with piercings that have grown over the years from small holes to long, vertical lines.

Technique: Performed with a local or topically applied anaesthetic, if the earlobe is newly split, the surgeon will simply stitch it up. If the lobe has been split in the past and

healed itself, or if you want to correct the elongated, vertical line, a piece of skin will be cut out to obtain a raw edge that the surgeon will then stitch. Both procedures take less than half an hour to perform.
Downtime: None.
Complications: The earlobe is one of the most common parts of the body to develop keloid scars, which are thick, red, and raised. There is also a small risk of infection, and the ear should not be re-pierced on the incision for at least three months.
Post-treatment: There may be some discomfort for a few days and a pain medication such as Tylenol can be taken. Avoid touching the lobe or putting any excess pressure on it.
Results: A ripped earlobe will be repaired, and/or the elongated vertical holes caused by the wearing of heavy earrings will be removed.
Ideal Candidate: If your lobe has been accidentally torn, or if you have piercings that have become elongated over the years, you are a definite candidate for this surgery.
How Often: Once.
Cost: $500 to $100 per year

Prominent Ears Correction (Otoplasty)

Background: The second type of surgery is performed to correct ears that appear to be too large because they do not fold back. This folding back process is one of the last events to happen while we are still in our mother's womb, but in approximately 2 percent of the population, this normal growth stage does not occur. Most often the defect is corrected in childhood, when the child is over the age of five and the ear has reached 85 percent of its growth. However, the surgery, which entails recreating the fold and pulling the ear back to make it less prominent, can also be performed on adults.
Technique: Considered to be intricate surgery, the procedure is done either under a local anaesthetic with an intravenous

sedation or under a general anaesthetic in a hospital or a clinic. Taking about one to two hours, the surgeon will first make an incision on the back of the ear. Then the natural fold is recreated either with stitches, or by attempting to re-bend the fold. Sometimes cartilage is weakened through a scoring technique and combined with sutures. The bowl of the ear will often be pulled back in the process. A turban like bandage, which will ward off swelling and hold everything in place, will then be applied.

Downtime: One to two weeks.

Complications: There will be some swelling and mild discomfort for at least a week. There is also the risk of infection and blood clots or hematomas forming under the skin. Because the cartilage is very sensitive, infection and/or bleeding can cause permanent damage, resulting in misshaped cartilage. Keloid scar formation and having ears that are not perfectly symmetrical with each other are also possible risks. In approximately less than 5 percent of all cases, and mostly in adults (since the cartilage has more memory), the newly shaped ear will unfold, and another operation will be required.

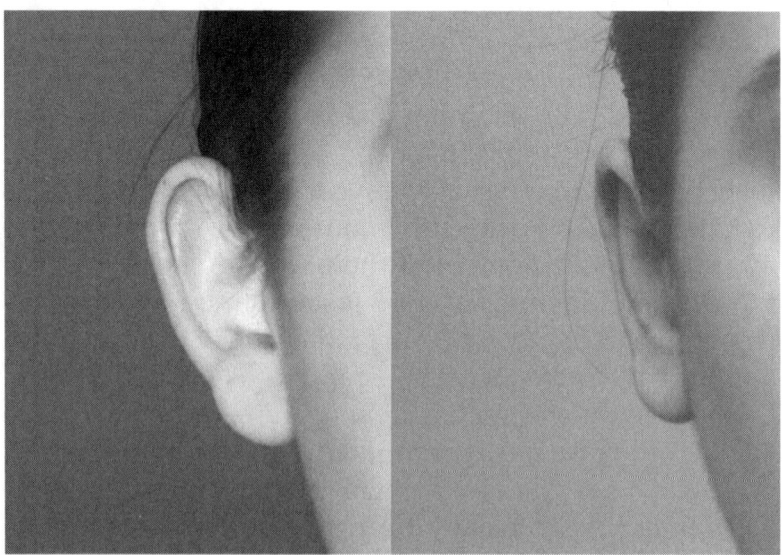

Correction of prominent ears with otoplasty.

Chapter 9| Facial Contouring

Post-treatment: Excessive pain medication is to be avoided after this operation, especially in children, because if a blood clot is forming the associated pain would alert the surgeon, who can act immediately to correct it. Adults may take Tylenol 3 if absolutely necessary. The bandages will come off after a week; however, a headband should be worn to protect the ears for another couple of weeks. When the bandages come off, you may wash your hair with a gentle shampoo. Avoid any heavy exercise or any situation where the ear may accidentally be hit or pulled forward for at least three weeks.

Results: Large, prominent ears that stick out from the head will appear smaller, less noticeable, tucked in, or pinned back.

Ideal Candidate: This operation is ideally suited to children five years of age and older, whose ears have not folded back. If you are an adult with the same condition, you are also a candidate; however, there is a slightly increased chance that the operation may have to be redone.

How Often: This operation should only have to be performed once, unless complications arise, which could mean a second operation.

Cost: $4,000–$5,000.

MOST COMMONLY ASKED QUESTIONS

Question: I'm nervous about having silicone in my body. What are the facial implants usually made of?

Answer: The implants are typically formed from silicone. However, there has never been a correlation between solid silicone implants and any autoimmune disease (see Chapter 12, "Breast Enhancements").

Question: My ears stick out, but I have heard that I should have had surgery when I was a child to correct this. Can I still have it performed?

Answer: Although ear surgery is usually performed on children after the age of five, adults can also have an otoplasty to correct ears that do not fold back properly.

Question: Can the ethnic appearance of a nose be changed?
Answer: African and Asian noses lack a strong nasal bridge (called the dorsum) and will usually require some sort of augmentation or support to be added. If you are interested in this type of surgery, ensure that your surgeon has experience with this type of nose reshaping.

Question: Are there any alternatives to facial implants for the cheek and chin?
Answer: Sometimes various fillers or your own fat can be used for a subtle change rather than using an implant (see Chapter 6, "Wrinkles").

Chapter 10

Body
Contouring

Gaining weight as we get older is a natural process of aging. Indeed, after we celebrate our thirty-fifth or fortieth birthday, most of us tend to put on an additional 4.5 kilograms of weight for each decade until we reach sixty-five, when it gradually begins to fall off. And during the menopause period of a woman's life, she will usually notice an even bigger jump in her weight. While this weight gain is normal to the majority of us, it can usually be kept under control with a healthy lifestyle. Nevertheless, due to genetic disposition, there is a certain segment of the population that will be in relatively good physical shape but will have a localized area on their body that does not respond to any form of diet or exercise. Whether it be a large stomach, heavy thighs, or a double chin, these confined areas of excess fat can cause an enormous amount of frustration.

Liposuction, or the surgical removal of fat using suction devices, is one of the most popular ways to treat this unwanted fat in certain areas of the body, and is often performed in conjunction with other cosmetic surgeries such as a facelift or abdominoplasty, which is more commonly known as a tummy tuck (see Chapter 11, "Surgical Lifting for the Body"). Although many people believe that liposuction is a weight-loss procedure, it is actually designed to re-contour the problem area. In fact, most physicians will turn you away if you are looking to lose kilograms from your overall body weight.

Although some research indicates that liposuction may increase metabolism and therefore may be of benefit to the obese, the procedure is not generally done on anyone who is grossly overweight. Instead, it is a procedure ideally suited to a healthy person of close to normal weight.

LIPOSUCTION (TRADITIONAL/ TUMESCENT/ULTRASONIC)

Background: One of today's most popular cosmetic procedures, liposuction has come a long way since it was first performed in 1921 on a ballerina's knees. Crudely performed, and without the benefit of antibiotics, this primitive operation resulted in severe and permanent injury to both of the ballerina's legs. Over the ensuing decades, there wasn't much advancement in the method of surgery as physicians attempted to remove excess fat by cutting the skin, scraping the fat out with an instrument, and then utilizing some type of suction device to clean the area of any remnants of fat. This coarse technique was fraught with skin healing problems, scarring, bleeding, and infections.

It wasn't until 1975 when an Italian father-and-son team of doctors named Fischer developed what is now called the traditional method of liposuction, whereby small, blunt-tipped tubes (called cannulas) are inserted into the skin by way of tiny incisions. The tubes vary in size, depending on the area being liposuctioned. Under the chin, for example, where the fat is more watery in texture, a finer tube would be used than one on the abdomen, where the fat is denser in consistency. The physician moves the cannula around

Chapter 10| Body Contouring

under the skin, and either manually using a syringe, or by a way of a power device that produces suction, removes the subcutaneous fat. Although there were less scars and healing problems associated with traditional liposuction, bleeding, pain, and a high risk of infection still persisted.

Then in 1987, a dermatologist by the name of Jeffrey Klein revolutionized the entire procedure by developing what is known as tumescent liposuction. By injecting lidocaine (a local anaesthetic), epinephrine (also known as adrenaline, to shrink capillaries), and sometimes including cortisone (to control inflammation), and bicarbonate (to ease the pain of the injections) into a saline solution prior to traditional liposuction, the overall procedure was dramatically improved. Reacting to the huge amount of solution that is injected into the body through the tumescent method, the fat layer expands and becomes firmer, allowing the cannula to move more precisely under the skin. As blood vessels spasm and shrink with the introduction of the epinephrine to the solution, bleeding during the operation is minimal. The lidocaine sometimes precludes a general anaesthetic from being administered, while the cortisone curbs inflammation and subsequent swelling.

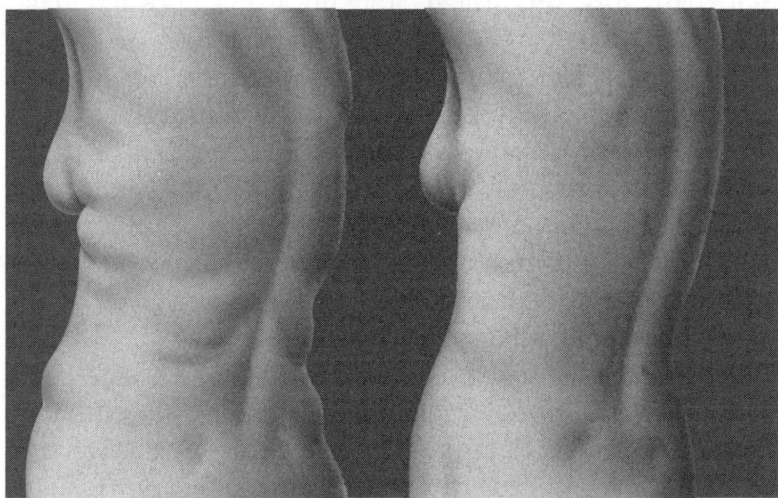

Drawings of a woman's torso before and after liposuction.

The ratio of fluid injected to the amout of fluid and fat removed varies from surgeon to surgeon.

The next breakthrough in liposuction came about in 1992, when another Italian, by the name of Dr. Zocchi, introduced the ultrasonic technique. This method uses energy produced by sound waves, which are set at a certain frequency and are passed into the fat via the cannula. The sound waves then break down the fat cells, melting or liquefying them before they are sucked out. This method results in less damage to blood vessels and nerves, thereby reducing the amount of swelling, bleeding, and bruising. However, because the energy was so difficult to control, there were numerous problems, such as burns, loss of skin, and infection associated with the ultrasonic technique, and it fell out of favour until 1997, when modifications were made to the system. Currently ultrasonic liposuction is much more controlled, but the American Society for Aesthetic Plastic Surgery recommends that only those physicians who have taken a training course should use it in their practice. It is of particular benefit if large volumes of fat are to be liposuctioned or for high resistant areas of fat that are more fibrous in their consistency, such as the back, sides, male breasts, and male "love handles." Still, many surgeons disagree that ultrasonic liposuction has any added benefit over traditional liposuction.

Another adjunct to liposuction evolved from the ultrasonic technique and is called external ultrasound-assisted liposuction (EUAL). By applying ultrasound to the outside of the skin before performing liposuction, it was thought that the fat would break down and become softer. Supposedly there would be less pain, swelling, and bruising after surgery. However, even though this is used in many practices, there is no strong clinical proof that it is of any significant benefit whatsoever.

Technique: Performed in a hospital on an "out-patient" basis, or a clinic, traditional liposuction will take approximately one to two hours to complete, while ultrasonic liposuction can take longer. Because the pre-treatment injection of fluids (e.g. tumescent liposuction) is so advantageous, it is now

Chapter 10| **Body Contouring** 145

almost always performed before either traditional or ultrasonic liposuction. However, depending on the volume of fat being removed, and the type of liposuction you are having, you may be given either a local anaesthetic along with an intravenous sedation, or a general anaesthetic.

Tiny incisions will be made and long needles will then be inserted to inject the tumescent fluids into the subcutaneous fat layer. After this has been completed, a waiting period of approximately ten to fifteen minutes is required to allow the fluids to penetrate the fat. Then a suction cannula is inserted to remove the fat. This cannula will either have a syringe on the end, which will allow the doctor to manually operate the cannula, or it will be hooked up to a vacuum or power suction device.

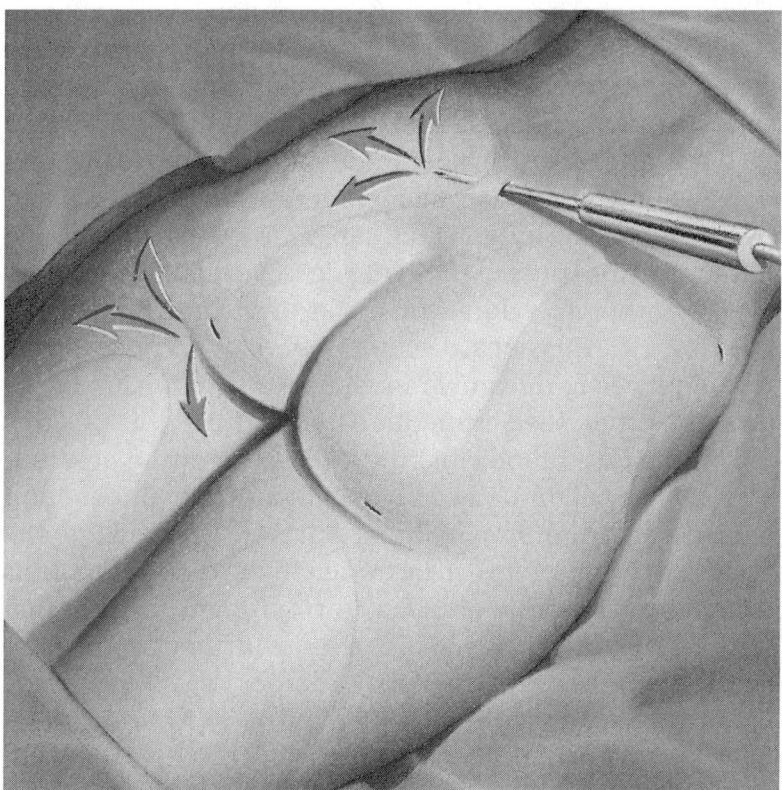

Drawing of the liposuction procedure being performed on a woman's buttocks and hips.

Approximately five to six litres of fat and fluids (which were introduced to your body during the tumescent procedure) will be removed during the liposuction. Any more than this amount is considered to be large-volume liposuction and should be avoided since it is associated with higher risks.

Once the liposuction has been completed, absorbent pads may be placed over the incisions, which may or may not be sutured, and will allow any excess fluid to drain. The pads will be held in place by wearing a compression garment over the area. For example, if you have had liposuction performed on your thighs, you will leave the clinic wearing a garment that looks like a pair of bicycle shorts.

Downtime: Two to four days.

Complications: Immediate, but uncommon, concerns associated with liposuction include complications with local or general anaesthetic; excessive fluid shifts in the body which can cause rapid changes in blood pressure and lead to a strain on the heart; excessive bleeding and thus a need for a blood transfusion and its associated problems, and the risk of fat or blood clots to the lungs which can interfere with breathing. Although rare, some of these risks can be fatal.

After the procedure, you can expect some drainage of fluid from the incisions, discomfort, swelling, and bruising. If you notice significantly more pain or swelling in one leg than the other, seek immediate medical attention, as this may indicate a blood clot. There is also a strong possibility that you will initially gain weight after the liposuction because of the amount of fluids that were injected into the body. This weight gain can be evident for up to three months afterwards. There may also be slight asymmetry in areas that were liposuctioned, which may require further treatment to correct. Numbness of the skin is another risk, however, the majority of patients will get the feeling back in the areas that have been liposuctioned within one year. Skin loss or skin sloughing is possible, but is extremely rare. Further and later complications are the possibility of raised, red hypertrophic

Chapter 10| **Body Contouring** 147

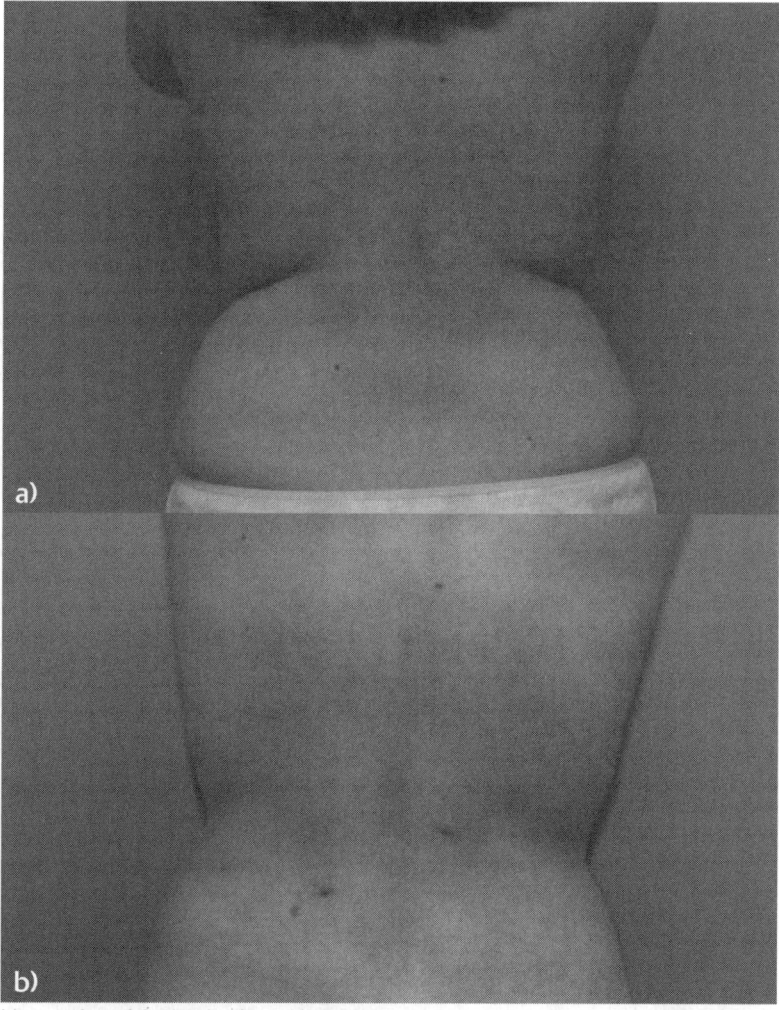
Liposuction of the back. a) pre b) post

scars that can be visible, especially around the knee area, and irregularities and rippling under the skin. How much your skin will tighten or contract won't be apparent for approximately one year after liposuction. If the skin is too loose, another operation to remove excess skin may be required.

Post-treatment: One of the most important things you must do after liposuction is to drink plenty of fluids to help replace the fluids leaking from the liposuctioned areas. For any mild aches and pains that you may experience, you can take a medication such as Tylenol 3.

The compression garment must be worn for four to six weeks; however, on the third day after liposuction, you may remove it to take a shower. Although you may begin moderate exercise twenty-four hours after the procedure, any heavy exercise should not be resumed for at least one month.

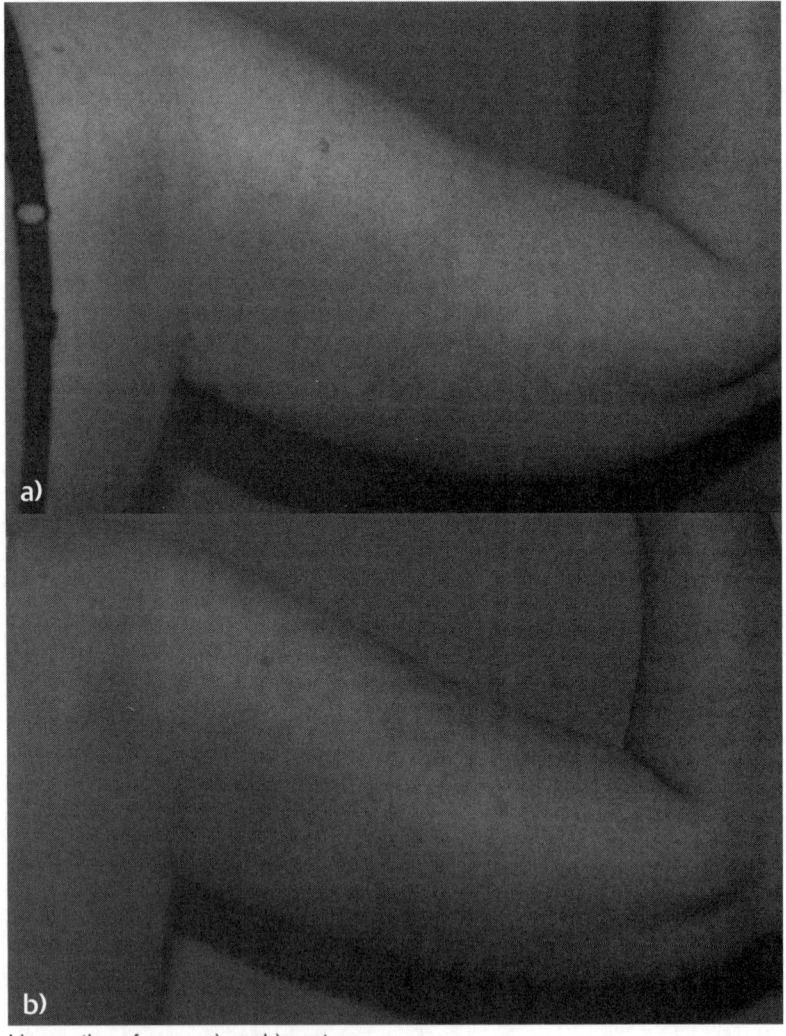

Liposuction of arms. a) pre b) post

Results: Do not expect to lose weight or cure cellulite from this operation. Instead, the targeted areas of fat will be reduced, resulting in a re-contouring of the body.

Ideal Candidate: If you are healthy, in good physical shape and close to a normal weight, but cannot reduce fat in certain areas of your body no matter how much you diet or exercise, liposuction may be of benefit.

How Often: Once, unless there are asymmetrical problems, which may have to be corrected, or if more than five litres of fat and fluid have to be removed, in which case a second liposuction will be required.

Cost: $3,500–$4,500 for one main area; $3,500 for under the chin; $1,000 for each additional area. Additional costs will be incurred if the procedure is done under general anaesthetic.

MESOTHERAPY

Background: Developed by Dr. Pistor in 1952, and given formal recognition by the French Academy of Medicine in 1987, mesotherapy is a technique that involves injecting a mixture of vitamins, amino acids, homeopathic medication, and other medications under the skin (mesoderm), to block our ability to store fat and stimulate the rate at which we burn it up. Presently used in Europe, Great Britain, and South America, this procedure has only recently been introduced to the North American market. Mesotherapy is most often used by those persons who may find liposuction too invasive or for those who have already had liposuction but have other fat deposits that have built up over a period of time. It is particularly beneficial in reducing isolated pockets of fats, such as what is commonly known as "love handles" or "saddlebags."

Technique: Taking only minutes to complete, you will be given several small injections of the mixture.

Downtime: Little or none.

Complications: There may be some redness, mild swelling, itchiness, and bruising in the treated areas, which will subside in a few days.

Post-treatment: You may apply ice or cold packs to the injected areas to minimize the associated redness and swelling.
Results: Over the course of several treatments, the skin will appear more toned as the fat in the injected areas lessens.
Ideal Candidate: If you have small localized areas of excess fat, you may be a good candidate for this therapy.
How Often: Ten sessions of injections per treated area will be required.
Cost: $200–$400 per session.

MOST COMMONLY ASKED QUESTIONS

Question: I have heard that once cells are liposuctioned, they disappear and never regrow. Is this true?
Answer: The fat cells that are removed by liposuction do not grow back. However, the remaining fat cells can compensate and grow larger if there is weight gain or changes in behavioural patterns, such as a decrease in exercise and increase in calorie intake.
Question: I'm overweight. Will liposuction make me lose weight?
Answer: There have been studies done on obese patients who have had large volume liposuction, which seem to indicate an association between the procedure and an increase in metabolism. However, the risk factors associated with such a procedure are very high and therefore, this is not a standard of care. Liposuction is better used on localized areas for someone who is maintaining their weight through good health and exercise.
Question: Will I be left with loose skin after liposuction?
Answer: Although liposuction does not tighten the skin, after time and healing some contraction of the skin will usually occur, especially in younger patients. It may take one year to see the final result.
Question: Will I need liposuction again?
Answer: Areas that have been treated will usually remain the same, unless there are significant changes in body weight.

Chapter 10| **Body Contouring** 151

Question: I hate exercising. Can I have liposuction instead?
Answer: No surgical procedure is a replacement for good health and exercise. When combined with a healthy lifestyle, liposuction can give excellent results. Liposuction alone will not treat the underlying problem or cause of the patient's unhappiness with their body shape and size.

Question: I have thick calves. Can they be liposuctioned?
Answer: Liposuction can be done on the calves, however, only a small volume of fat can be removed. This procedure will not change the underlying anatomy, bony structure, or muscular structure of your body. It will only treat the layer of fat between the skin and muscle.

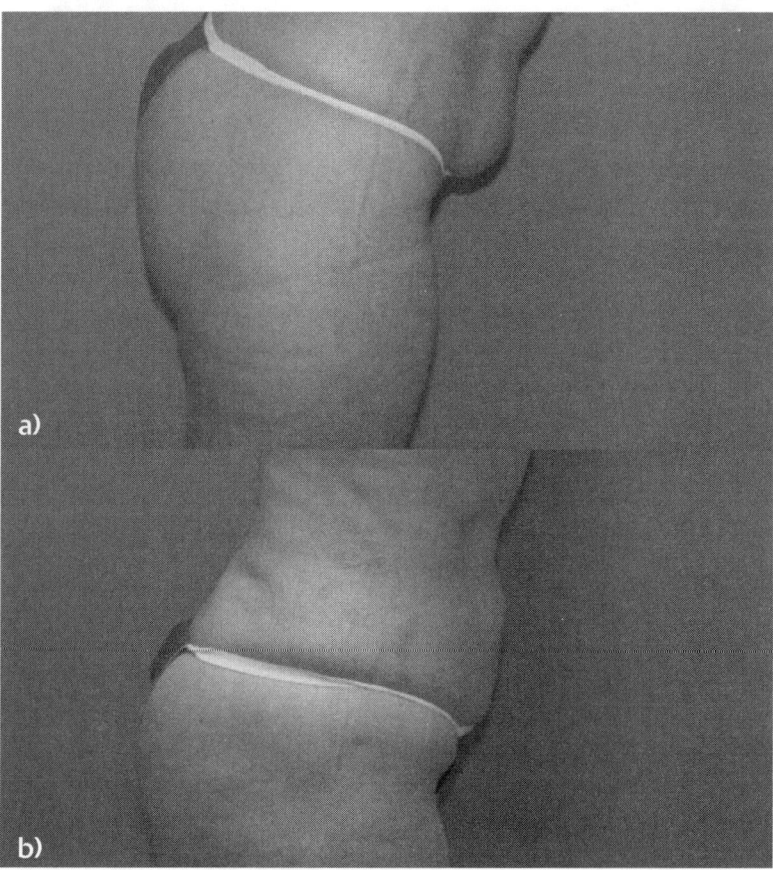

Liposuction of the abdomen. a) pre b) post

Chapter 11

Surgical Lifting
for the Body

You've been on a diet for the last twelve months, carefully measuring each gram of fat, carbohydrate, or calorie intake. Twice a week, you've visited the gym, where you used the various apparatus and took an aerobics class for good measure. And every morning, you've done fifty "crunches" to improve your abdomen, thirty "donkey-kicks" to get rid of the fat on your thighs, and a combination of other exercises in your continuous battle of the bulge. One morning, you step on the scales and are overjoyed to see that you've finally reached your goal. At long last, your weight is down. But as you look in the mirror, your happiness may be short-lived.

If you're like most people who have had a significant decrease in their weight, you may notice loose skin hanging like a doughy apron from your waist. Your rear end may appear as deflated as a half-filled balloon, and the skin on your middle or outer thighs may look so droopy you're seriously considering never wearing a pair of shorts again.

And then there's the loose skin that just seems to get worse as we age. Especially that floppy piece that dangles under our upper arms, making us look as if we're ready to take flight. No matter how thin we are, or how many weights we lift, it seems to have a life of its own, and only gets worse with time. And we thought those "bat-wings" were only supposed to happen to our grannies. Well, think again. The reality is, as we get older, our skin loses its elasticity. Compound that with weight loss, multiple surgeries, and pregnancies and other hormonal changes, and the result can be flaccid, limp skin.

The good news is this laxity can be improved with a variety of surgical lifting techniques. Whether it be an abdominoplasty that will remove excess skin from your waistline, a brachioplasty to reduce the skin on your upper arms, a thigh or buttock lift, modern surgical procedures can drastically revamp the shape and contour of your body.

TUMMY TUCK (ABDOMINOPLASTY)

Background: The first transverse removal of skin and fat for cosmetic purposes is attributed to a surgeon by the name of Kelly, who performed the operation at John Hopkins University in 1889. This early surgery simply involved cutting away excess skin on the abdomen. Thereafter, improvements in the abdominoplasty or tummy tuck procedure, as it is more commonly known, came about very slowly, and it wasn't until 1967 that a Brazilian surgeon named Pitanguay, developed the technique that lifted the skin around the navel, which was left intact, cut away the excess, and then pulled the skin above the navel downward. By stretching the skin, strengthening the underlying muscle, hiding the scar, and not sacrificing the navel, which had previously been cut away, Dr. Pitanguay lay the foundation for the modern-day abdominoplasty.

Currently there are several options available to excise or tighten loose skin on the abdomen. You may choose

Chapter 11| Surgical Lifting for the Body

liposuction (see Chapter 10, "Body Contouring"); a mini-abdominoplasty with liposuction, which only corrects the loose skin below the navel; a "floating belly-button" technique, which addresses the excess skin below the navel and a small amount above it; a reverse abdominoplasty, which only treats the skin above the navel; or a full abdominoplasty, which deals with the entire abdomen from the top of the rib cage to the pubic bone.

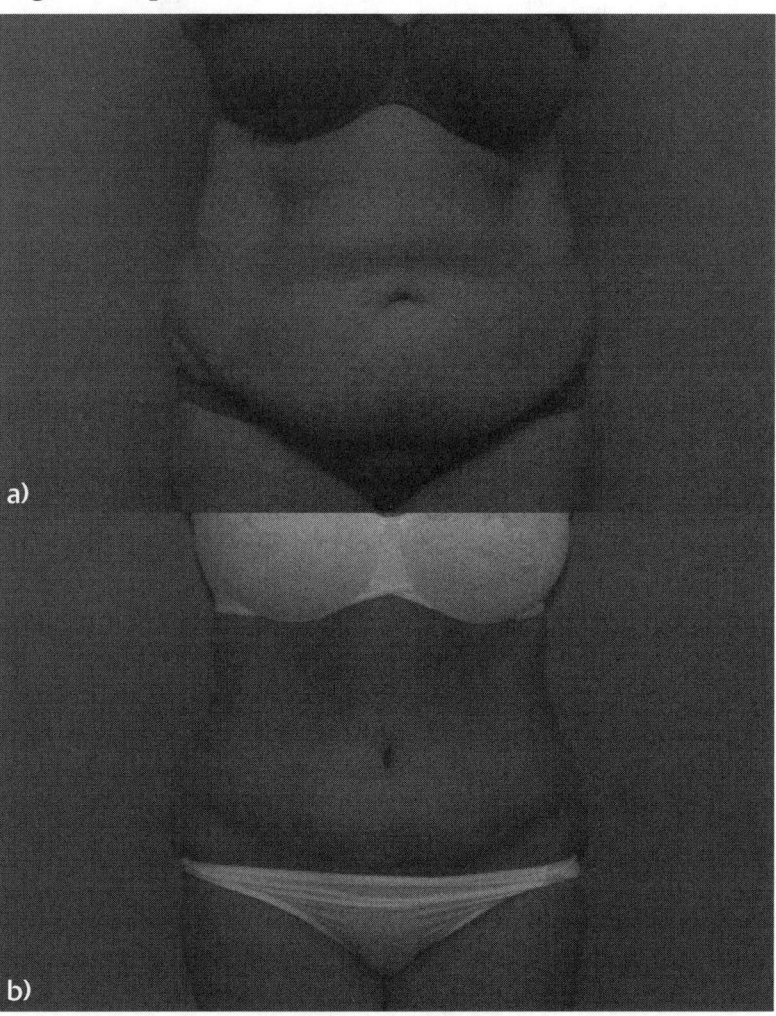

Abdominoplasty. a) pre b) four weeks postop (the red scar will fade with time)

A tummy tuck can be performed in combination with a medial (middle inside) or lateral (outside) thigh lift, especially in those people who have had a significant drop in weight, and a breast lift, reduction, or augmentation (see Chapter 12, "Breast Enhancements"). In some cases, it is also done in conjunction with surgery such as a hysterectomy. However, many surgeons prefer not to combine too many procedures because of the extended time it will take to operate, resulting in higher risks associated with being under a general anaesthetic for too long. Infections are also more common in compounded procedures, especially if the tummy tuck is being done at the same time as gynecological surgery.

As with any cosmetic surgery, you must first consult with a qualified surgeon, who will determine what type of operation is required. During this initial consultation, the physician will discuss your exercise and diet habits and determine whether your weight is stable and whether or not you have had previous abdominal surgery, pregnancies, or significant changes in your weight. Your health history, which can affect the risk of complications during and after the operation, will also be discussed. (Diabetics and smokers are at the highest risk.) Then your surgeon will examine you while you are standing, to get a sense of how lax the abdominal muscles are. Next, you will be asked to sit down, which will give the physician an idea of how much loose skin there is above and below the navel. You will also be asked to perform half of a sit-up, which will allow the surgeon to determine how far apart your abdominal muscles are spread. Then, by having you lie down, the physician will assess the amount of intra-abdominal fat you have and get a further sense of what the end result of the operation will be.

This is also a good test to give yourself before considering an abdominoplasty. If, when you lie down, you like the results, then you may be a good candidate. If you are still unhappy about the shape of your abdomen, you should know that your surgeon cannot improve it beyond the way it looks when you

Chapter 11| Surgical Lifting for the Body

are in a supine position. The fullness of the abdomen when you are lying down is contributed by intra-abdominal fat, bowels, and other organs. The only way to treat this type of persistent bulge is weight loss and exercise first. Finally, your doctor will give you an abdominal examination, which will ensure that nothing medical, such as a tumour, is causing the problem.

Technique: Performed in a clinic or a hospital, and under a general anaesthetic, a full abdominoplasty will usually require you to be in the clinic or hospital overnight, or as an outpatient, depending on your health history. If you are having a mini-abdominoplasty, a local anaesthetic with intravenous sedation may suffice. Other than this, and a few other minor variances, all of the levels of tummy tucks will be performed in much the same manner, and will only differ in the extent of how much skin is being cut, lifted, and re-draped. However, you should remember that surgeons have their own individual techniques, and operations may not be performed in the same exact manner as outlined below.

Antibiotics will be introduced into your system by way of intravenous (common to any surgery performed under a general anaesthetic), then a catheter will be inserted to deflate the bladder and keep it away from the area of operation. The catheter, which may be left in for the first twelve hours after the procedure, also allows the surgeon to monitor the fluid levels in your body. If the operation is being performed under a local, a catheter may not be necessary. You will also be given blood thinners and outfitted with thrombotic leg stockings or serial compression stockings that will continually massage the legs during the operation to help prevent deep vein thrombosis (blood clots).

For a full abdominoplasty, the initial incision will be made from hip bone to hip bone, under the roll of excess skin. The fat and skin layer above the muscle wall will then be lifted. Once this is complete, an incision will be made around the navel, leaving it attached to the muscle wall. The dissection will then continue up to the rib cage, just under the breasts. The bed is then flexed into a chair-like position and the access skin is removed. The underlying muscle will be sutured together and tightened, working like an internal girdle, which will often result in a cinching of the waistline. During this operation the contents of the abdomen will not be touched. Then the skin will be stretched downward to the pubic bone, and another incision will be made in the stretched skin for the navel. The operation will be closed with absorbable sutures under the skin, which will not require removal.

Before finishing the tummy tuck, tubes will usually be inserted into the abdomen to allow any fluids to drain, and a dressing will be placed over the tubes. These tubes may or may not be removed before you are discharged. In order to prevent pockets of fluids (called seromas), or blood (called hematomas) from forming between the muscle and skin wall, some surgeons will stitch the walls together in an attempt to obliterate the space between them. Finally, you will be placed in a compression garment like a girdle, which will support the area and also help to prevent seroma and hematoma formation.

Downtime: One to two weeks.

Complications: There are the usual risks associated with a general anaesthetic. Occurring in less than 1 out of 50,000 patients, they can include an allergy to the anaesthetic, adverse reactions, breathing and heart problems, and an abnormal rise in body temperature. There is also an occasional risk of bleeding, and an even lessor chance that you may require a transfusion. (There is also the chance of infection, and of a seroma or hematoma formation, which may have to be drained more than once with a needle.) The biggest danger, however, is that blood may pool in the legs, clot, break up, and travel to the lungs, which potentially can be fatal. The risk of deep vein thrombosis (DVT) is at its highest level three days after the operation, which is why it is vital that you are up and walking the day after your surgery. The risk

Chapter 11| Surgical Lifting for the Body 159

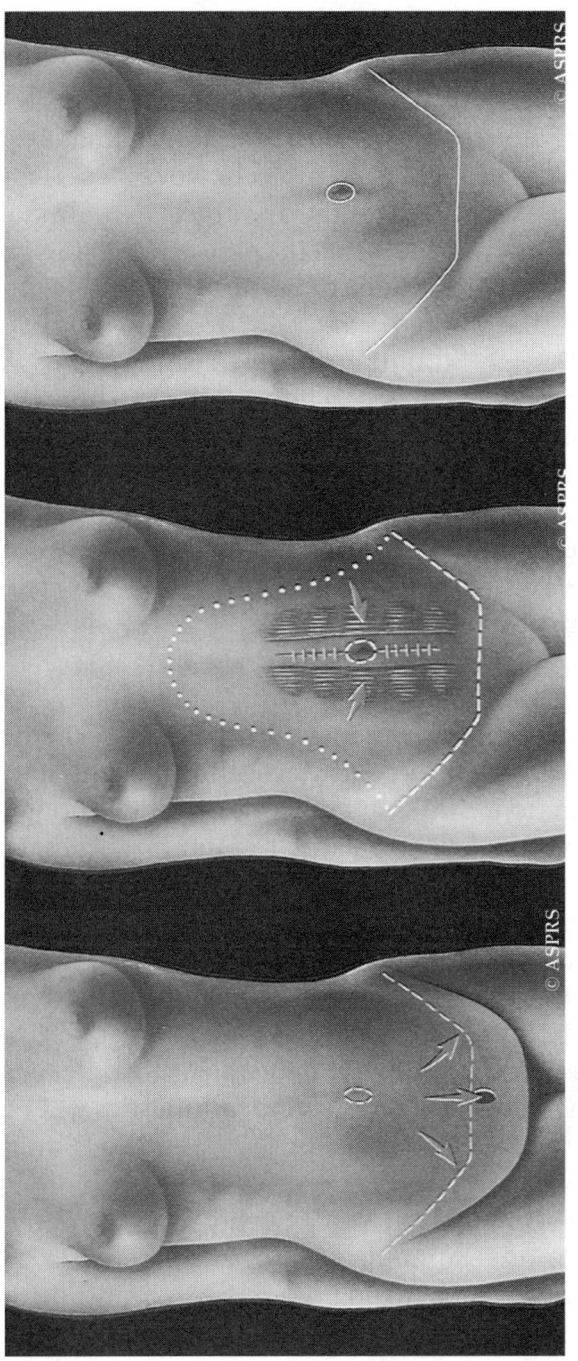

a) A skin incision is made under the lowest roll of excess skin.

b) The skin is lifted off the abdominal wall all the way to the rib cage. The excess skin is removed and the underlying muscles are sewn together like an internal girdle.

c) A new incision is made in the stretched skin for the belly button. All the incisions are closed.

of DVT is the highest with large orthopedic surgeries, such as hip replacement, but can occur after any surgical procedure. You will be quite sore in the abdomen area, and will be walking and sleeping in a stooped position for approximately a week. Asymmetry of the area is possible; however, less than 5 percent of patients require a touch-up surgery. Numbness or a loss of feeling to the skin will occur to almost all patients after the operation, and less than 10 percent will be left with permanent numbness after a year.

If the blood supply around the navel for some reason is compromised, there is a low risk that the navel will get infected and/or slough off. This is seen most often in smokers and/or diabetics. A small amount of skin loss or wound breakdown in the middle of the scar that runs from both hips, can occur which can usually be healed with an antibiotic ointment, but may require a second surgery to correct the remaining scar. Ten to 15 percent of patients will develop a hypertrophic scar, which is raised, red, and ropey in texture.

Post-treatment: Immediately following the operation, and for several days afterwards, you must drink plenty of fluids. If you do not feel like eating a solid diet for the first couple of days, diet supplement drinks are recommended. Although you will be uncomfortable, it is also extremely important to get up and walk the first day in order to prevent blood clots from forming in the legs. Tylenol 3 can be taken to relieve soreness and pain. If you are taking a codeine-based medication, ensure that you eat fibre and drink plenty of water, since you will want to avoid "pushing" that can result from codeine-induced constipation. If your health history dictates that you are at a higher risk for infection, antibiotics will be prescribed for up to a week following the operation. Avoid smoking for six weeks afterwards.

The drains will be removed within twenty-four to seventy-two hours, and if nonabsorbable stitches were used to close the operation, they will be taken out approximately one to two weeks after the procedure. Once the drains have been removed, you can shower; however, you should take the following steps when removing your compression garment (which you will continue to wear for three to six weeks). Because the garment restricts the return of the blood to your heart, there is a good possibility that you may pass out when you first take the garment off—especially if you are stepping into a hot shower. Remove it when lying down, then sit up and wait a few moments. Stand up, and wait another few minutes before taking your shower. Although mild exercise such as walking is recommended, any heavy exercise or lifting should be avoided for at least four to six weeks.

Typically, your surgeon will see you three days after the operation, then after one week, two weeks, six weeks, six months, and a year following the operation. However, if you have any concerns, or abnormal swelling or pain (especially in the legs), do not hesitate to immediately seek medical attention.

Results: Prior to the operation, lie down on a flat surface. The way you look in this position will dictate how you will look after the procedure in the standing position. Most of the excess skin will be removed, and your abdomen will be firmer and tighter.

Ideal Candidate: If you have loose skin and muscle laxity above or below the navel, caused from weight loss, pregnancies, or multiple surgeries, you may be a good candidate for this surgery. By taking the above-noted test prior to making a decision regarding this procedure, you can determine whether or not you are a candidate. If the stomach still protrudes when you are lying down, or if you are obese, this surgery is not for you. The only way to deal with internal abdominal fat is to lose weight, and then consider an abdominoplasty to deal with the loose, hanging skin and spread-out muscles. If you are considering further pregnancies, you should not get an abdominoplasty, since your skin stretch after surgery may decrease and also because further loose skin and muscle will likely reoccur after the pregnancy. Furthermore, although someone who has had multiple surgeries may be a good candidate because of the associated loose skin, if you have multiple scars in the area, they may interfere with the healing of the abdominoplasty wounds, and therefore you may not be suitable for this operation. A frank, open discussion with your surgeon will determine whether you should go ahead with a tummy tuck.

How Often: Once. If your weight remains normal, and you are in good health, other than obtaining a little more laxity as you age, you should not lose the initial result.

Cost: $7,500–$9,500 for a full abdominoplasty; $5,000–$6,000 for a mini-abdominoplasty.

MEDIAL ARM LIFT (BRACHIOPLASTY)

Background: According to statistics from the American Society for Aesthetic Plastic Surgery, upper arm reduction procedures increased by 321 percent since 1997. This heightened popularity can be attributed to the large number of people who have undergone modern gastrointestinal (bariatric) surgical procedures, such as stomach stapling or gastric banding performed through a scope, and have lost more than 45 kilograms (100 pounds) in weight. Indeed, many of these newly slimmed-down people often want their arms corrected before considering other skin-tightening operations. And while liposuction can remove any remaining fat, it will not deal with the loose skin that is the result of such a dramatic weight loss.

Another factor that is making brachioplasty more mainstream is that surgeons have refined the procedure, so that the resulting vertical scars are now placed so they cannot be seen while the arms are at rest. But there will still most definitely be a scar, and anyone contemplating a brachioplasty should take this into consideration. This operation is also deemed to be one that requires exceptional surgical skill and should only be performed by a qualified and certified surgeon (see Chapter 15, "Choosing A Qualified Specialist").

Chapter 11 | Surgical Lifting for the Body

Technique: Performed in a clinic or a hospital under a general anaesthetic, the operation may be conducted on an outpatient basis or may require an overnight stay. An incision may be made from the armpit area (called the axillia) along the underside of the arm to approximately the middle of the upper arm. Or if less skin excision is necessary a small horizontal scar in only the axilla may be used. If the procedure is being performed in conjunction with liposuction, as is often done, excess fat and skin will then be removed, with the surgeon being careful not to damage veins and superficial nerves. Drainage tubes may or may not be inserted. When the surgery is completed, you will most likely be outfitted with a pressure dressing.

Downtime: One to two weeks.

Complications: During surgery, there will be the potential risks associated with a general anaesthetic. There is also a danger of bleeding, blood clots, hematoma or seroma formation, and infection. Asymmetry of the two arms is possible and a touch-up surgery may be necessary. Expect some soreness and pain for the first couple of weeks after the procedure. Temporary numbness may also occur, and in some patients this may be permanent. Long, vertical scars, which may become raised red and thick hypertrophic scars, may also be visible when the arms are not in the resting position.

Post-treatment: Medication such as Tylenol 3 may be taken for any pain. Your compression dressing should be worn for several weeks after the surgery, including at night. Although mild exercise such as walking is recommended, any other aggressive physical exercise should be avoided for a month afterwards. If drainage tubes were inserted, they will be removed within twenty-four to seventy-two hours, and if nonabsorbable stitches were used, they will be taken out within ten days.

Results: The loose, hanging skin on the upper arms will be eliminated; however, there will be a noticeable scar when the arms are placed in certain positions.

Ideal Candidate: If you have flaccid skin that hangs from under the upper arms due to significant weight loss, hormonal changes, aging, or genetics and are willing to live with the scars that this operation will ensue, then you are a good candidate for a brachioplasty.
How Often: Once.
Cost: $5,500.

THIGH LIFT

Background: There are several ways to deal with loose skin on the thigh area: a medial lift, which corrects the middle inside of the thighs; a lateral lift, which addresses the outside of the thighs; a posterior lift for the back of the thighs; or a buttock lift.

Although the surgeon will attempt to hide the scars in the creases around the legs, there will be noticeable scars as a consequence of the various types of thigh lifts, and therefore the procedure is usually limited to post-bariatric patients who have lost at least 45 kilograms of weight as a result of surgery and those patients with significantly loose skin.

Technique: Often performed in conjunction with liposuction, this procedure will be done under a general anaesthetic in a clinic or hospital. Depending on your health history, you will either be admitted as an outpatient or you may require an overnight stay. You will be given blood thinners and most likely outfitted with thrombotic leg stockings or serial compression stockings that will massage the legs during the operation to help prevent blood clots from forming.

Incisions will be made depending on where the skin requires lifting. In most cases, surgeons will attempt to hide some of the scars by incising in the groin area; however, there will be other areas of incisions that will result in visible scars. After the incisions are made, the fat from the deeper muscle layers and the skin will be lifted and re-draped. Tubes that will drain any fluids may or may not be inserted. Once the operation is complete, you will be placed in a compression garment resembling bicycle shorts.

Chapter 11| **Surgical Lifting for the Body**   165

Downtime: One to two weeks.
Complications: During the operation, there is a rare risk of bleeding and other dangers associated with being under a general anaesthetic. There is also the possibility that blood clots may form. Because the risk of deep vein thrombosis is at its highest three days after the operation, it is imperative that you are up and walking the day following surgery. Expect some pain and soreness for a few days afterwards. Since some of the incisions will be made in the groin area, which is a moist environment, there is a higher risk of infection associated with this operation. Hematomas and seromas may also form. Asymmetry of the thighs is possible and may require a second surgery to correct. The greatest complications of this surgery are the visible scars, which may be raised, red, and thick in texture and incomplete removal of all the loose skin.
Post-treatment: Although you will be in moderate pain after the operation, it is vital that you get up and walk within a day. You can take Tylenol 3 to control the soreness and pain. If drains were inserted, they will be removed within twenty-four to seventy-two hours after surgery, and if the stitches used were nonabsorbable, they will be taken out approximately ten days after surgery. You should wear the compression garment for four to six weeks, but three days after the procedure you can remove it to take a shower.
Results: This operation will lift, tighten, and remove excess skin on the thigh area. However, scars will be visible.
Ideal Candidate: If you have lost in excess of 45 kilograms of weight as a result of bariatric surgery, you may be a good candidate for a thigh lift.
How Often: Once.
Cost: $5,500–$6,500.

BUTTOCK ENHANCEMENT

Background: The desire for a higher, fuller rear end has come in and out of style several times over the last century. Victorian women wore bustles to acquire the effect, and padded girdles were introduced in the 1950s. Currently, as a result of the popularity of some Latin female celebrities, having larger buttocks is back in fashion with the younger generation. Indeed, buttock augmentation and lifts are presently one of the most routine cosmetic procedures in Brazil, and are becoming more commonplace in North America, especially with anyone who has had a dramatic weight loss.

This fuller look to the rear end is sometimes achieved with the use of solid silicone implants. However, the operation will leave visible scars, and the implants will have a tendency to shift, which can require a second operation to correct. Gaining more popularity is a combination of skin lifting, in which incisions are made under the crease and excess skin is cut away, and the fat grafting technique, which involves taking fat from your own body through liposuction (see Chapter 10, "Body Contouring") and injecting it into the buttocks.

Technique: Depending on the type of operation being performed, you will be given either a general anaesthetic or a local with an intravenous sedation. The procedure will take place in a clinic or hospital and you will most likely be admitted as an outpatient. If liposuction is involved, fat will be taken from a donor site in your body and injected into each side of the buttock through two small criss-cross entry points. If implants are being inserted, they will require larger incisions to create a pocket for the implants. These procedures may or may not be combined with lifting, cutting, and re-draping of excess skin, which will require incisions either under the buttock crease or on the upper aspect of the buttocks. When the operation is completed, drainage tubes may or may not be inserted, and you will be outfitted with a compression garment.

Downtime: One to two weeks.

Complications: If the procedure was done under a general anaesthetic there will be the usual dangers associated with it. Bleeding, blood clots, and infection are also possibilities. Expect to be in some pain afterwards. Nerve injury is rare but can occur. If implants are inserted, there is a possibility they

Chapter 11| Surgical Lifting for the Body

will shift and require a second surgery to correct. Implants and lifting will result in visible scars, which can become hypertrophic (i.e., raised, red thick scars).

Post-treatment: Pain medication such as Tylenol 3 can be taken. It is important to be up and walking a day after surgery to lessen the risk of blood clots. If drains were inserted, they will be removed twenty-four to seventy-two hours afterwards, while nonabsorbable sutures will be taken out within ten days. Wear your compression garment for six weeks, and leave it on for three days before removing it for the first time to shower. Avoid any strenuous activity for at least a month. For the first few days it is recommended to avoid sitting and sleep on your front.

Results: Implants and fat grafting will achieve a fuller, rounder look to the buttocks, while skin lifting will remove and tighten any loose, excess skin.

Ideal Candidate: If you have had a dramatic weight loss and have flaccid, hanging skin in the buttock area, or have a flat rear end due to genetics, you may be a good candidate for the surgeries.

How Often: Once.
Cost: $5,000–$7,000.

MOST COMMONLY ASKED QUESTIONS

Question: What can I expect when I get a tummy tuck?
Answer: When you lie down and look at your abdomen, you will see much the same as a tummy tuck can do. If you still have a very protuberant stomach when lying down, this is probably due to intra-abdominal fat, which will not be treated with an abdominoplasty.

Question: I've had multiple pregnancies, and even though I exercise, I still have loose skin on my stomach. Am I candidate for a tummy tuck?
Answer: The main procedure involved in an abdominoplasty is the removal of loose skin. You may be very thin and in excellent shape, but cannot regain the elasticity of your skin after

giving birth or if you've had a significant previous weight loss. Exercise alone or liposuction will not help. However, excising the skin will give you a much tighter, flatter abdomen.

Question: Can I combine my tummy tuck with other surgeries?

Answer: You must be aware that the more surgeries you combine, the higher the risk of infection. As well, there is an increased risk of bleeding and blood clots forming in the legs due to the increased length of time while in surgery.

Question: I am very skinny. Does that mean I will only need a mini tummy tuck?

Answer: A mini tummy tuck is defined by the correction of the loose skin of the abdomen solely below the navel. Therefore, you may or may not require a full or a mini tummy tuck, and this will be assessed by your doctor upon examination.

Question: Can I have my hips and thighs liposuctioned at the same time as my tummy tuck?

Answer: Most often, a small amount of liposuction is performed at the time of the tummy tuck, particularly in the flank and hip area. However, aggressive liposuction is not usually combined with a full abdominoplasty because of the associated increase risk of bleeding, prolonged healing time, risk of blood clots, and other complications.

Question: How much time off work is typically required following an abdominoplasty?

Answer: If you have a job that does not require any lifting, you can usually return to work after one to two weeks. However, if your job involves lifting, it is recommended that you take four to six weeks off.

Question: What is bariatric surgery?

Answer: This is gastrointestinal surgery that involves stomach stapling or gastric banding performed through a scope and is performed on those who are obese, requiring at least a 45-kilogram weight loss. Many of these patients will require further surgery once their weight loss has plateaued to remove the excess skin.

Chapter 12

Breast
Enhancements

The grass is always greener, they say, and this especially rings true when women think of their own breasts, which in our minds are either too big, too small, or too droopy. The woman with larger breasts longs for the day when her back no longer aches, or just to be able to participate in simple aerobic activity, while the smaller-breasted woman is frustrated with wearing padded brassieres to give her flatter chest a more shapely appearance. Even the woman who may have once had a "perfect" breast size before pregnancy is dissatisfied with the way her breasts now hang loosely against her abdomen.

Modern-day breast enhancement covers a wide array of surgeries that can correct these problems, either by making the breasts bigger through augmentation (augmentation mammoplasty), smaller through a breast reduction (reduction mastopexy), or perkier by way of a breast lift (mastoplexy). And while an augmentation, in which an implant is inserted into the breast to give it a fuller and larger look, may or may not be combined with a lift, when a breast is reduced in size it is also always lifted during the process. Covering a spectrum of procedures from liposuction to major surgery, the scope of a breast reduction or lift will depend on the desired results. Whatever your choice, the ensuing size and shape of your breasts can give you a better-proportioned figure and boost your self-esteem and confidence in the process.

Although breast lifts are often done on their own without reducing or increasing the size of the breast, as mentioned, the reduction is always done with a lift, and the techniques used for both operations are similar. As such, the mastopxy and reduction mammoplasty surgeries will be described under the same section below.

BREAST REDUCTION (REDUCTION MAMMOPLASTY) AND LIFT (MASTOPEXY)

Background: The first breast reduction for cosmetic purposes was performed in Paris in the late 1800s, and basically involved cutting a crescent-shaped piece of the breast away. Then in 1907, a similar procedure was done to correct asymmetry on a patient who had different sized breasts. A few years later another operation was devised, which dissected the breast off the muscle in an attempt to lift and reduce its size. By 1923, surgery to reduce or lift the breasts had evolved to making an incision (called an inverted T or an anchor incision) around the nipple, straight up and down under the nipple area, and then underneath the breast, whereby a wedge was cut out of the lower breast, which was then pushed upwards.

In this early period of breast enhancement operations, reshaping of the breast was a difficult concept for surgeons to understand. There was no real idea of how much skin to cut off, or how to re-drape it afterwards to give the breast a natural appearance. But in the 1930s, a surgeon had an epiphany and realized that the skin on the chest served as a

Chapter 12| Breast Enhancements

"brassiere" for the actual breast. Subsequently, he went to a bra-making factory to observe the various three-dimensional shapes of the garments. From this came a deeper understanding of how to make the breast look more natural, and various patterns to improve the shape of the enhanced breasts evolved. Then in the 1940s and '50s, other developments came about in that surgeons began to experiment with leaving the nipple attached to the breast tissue. By not compromising the blood supply to this area the nipple could retain more sensation, and the new procedure may even allow for the future ability to breast-feed.

By the mid-1950s, the lifting of breasts had become an accepted operation, and a surgeon by the name of Wise began to educate other surgeons on how to remove breast tissue and reshape it, using what it called a "Wise geometrical pattern," in a consistent and safe manner. The final incision was around the nipple, straight down and under the breast crease like an anchor.

Subsequently, a surgeon by the name of Lejour created another technique, which remains very popular because it eliminated the scar underneath the breast. The incision, which resembles a lollipop, runs around the nipple and down to the crease but does not extend along the fold.

Technique: There are a variety of ways to perform breast reductions and lifts. The less involved operations will only require a local anaesthetic with an intravenous sedation, while the larger procedures will necessitate a general. They can all be performed in either a clinic or hospital, and in most cases, will not require an overnight stay. Although nipple loss is rare, it is more prevalent in smokers, who will be asked to quit for six weeks prior to the operation and for six weeks afterwards.

The full spectrum of operations will be described ranging from the least involved to the most complex.

1. For the woman who has almost no droop to the breasts, but wants to lose some volume, and whose nipples are

sitting in a correct position, meaning they sit at the projected level of the crease of your breast or slightly higher, liposuction (see Chapter 10, "Body Contouring") is recommended. Only fat and some tissue will be removed, while the skin will not be touched.
2. For the woman who has a small amount of droop and also some excess volume, then incisions will be made just around the nipples. The breast size will be left the same, while the nipple will be lifted up one to two centimetres. This can also be combined with liposuction to remove some of the tissue.
3. For the woman who has moderate drooping to the breasts, the lollipop incision (described above) will be used with almost no excision of tissue, allowing the same volume to be maintained. If the breast size is to be reduced, this will be combined with cutting and liposuction.
4. For the woman whose breasts sag, with the nipples sitting low on the chest, and which also have a great amount of tissue, a full reduction using an anchor or lollipop incision will be performed. Liposuction is added as needed, especially for the side fullness under the arm area.
5. For the woman who requires a massive breast reduction grater than 2kg per breast, a free nipple graft may be necessary. The lower half of the breast will be excised and the nipple will be removed as a thin skin graft and reapplied to the desired position. The nipple will lose its duct connections and blood supply, and will be reattached as a graft. The nipple will be nonfunctional and have no feeling, and the woman will have lost the ability to breast-feed.

When the procedure is complete, which can take from one to three hours, tubes to drain fluids may or may not be inserted, and the various incisions may be taped. Afterwards you will wear either your own brassiere or a surgical bra.

Chapter 12| **Breast Enhancements** 173

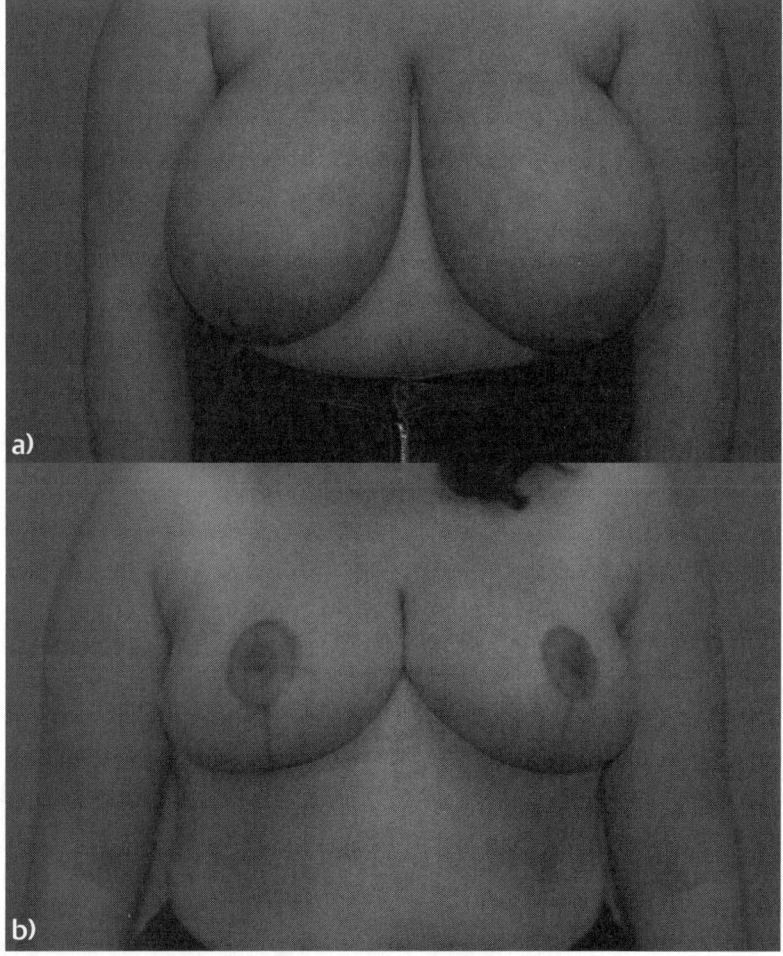

Breast reduction. a) pre b) early postop

Downtime: One to three weeks.
Complications: If performed under a general anaesthetic, there will be the usual associated risks. There may also be the chance of bleeding and the formation of deep vein blood clots. Less than 1 percent of patients will develop an infection. If a large amount of breast tissue has been removed, there is a risk that fluids can collect, which may have to be drained with a needle, or you may require a second operation. Depending on the procedure, there will be swelling, bruising, and some pain. There is also the danger

that the skin on the wounds may not heal properly. Because of the tension on the incisions, the breasts will be prone to hypertrophic or thick, red scars. Feeling in the nipples will be increased, decreased, or completely eliminated, and may also vary in each of the breasts. Asymmetry between the two breasts is very common pre-surgery, but can also arise following the operation and may require a second surgery to correct.

Because it is impossible for a surgeon to predict whether a woman will be able to breast-feed after a reduction or lift, it should be assumed that breast-feeding will not be an option afterwards. There is also no guarantee that back pain will decrease after a breast reduction, since damage to the back may already have been done. After either a reduction or a lift, there is no increase or decrease in the risk of breast cancer.

Post-treatment: Medication such as Tylenol 3 can be taken for any pain associated with the various procedures. If the skin on the wounds is not healing properly, an antibiotic ointment will be prescribed. Drains will be removed approximately twenty-four hours, while nonabsorbable sutures will be taken out within ten days. Since your blood count may drop slightly during and after the operation, you may not feel well for approximately one week after the procedure, however it is important that you are up and walking on the same day to avoid blood clots in the legs. Taking iron and vitamins after surgery can help with the problem. You may shower after the drains have been removed.

Results: Breasts will either be lifted or reduced in size and volume, giving the figure a more proportionate shape.

Ideal Candidate: If you are over the age of eighteen (when breast development has stopped), and have mild to severe drooping of the breasts or extremely large breasts, you will most likely benefit from the various procedures.

How Often: Once. However, changes in the breast may occur because of pregnancy, major weight shifts, menopause, and a further surgery may be required.

Cost: $6,000–$7,000.

BREAST AUGMENTATION (AUGMENTATION MAMMOPLASTY)

Background: For the past several decades, physicians and scientists have been attempting to create the perfect substance to inject or implant into a woman's breasts to increase their volume. The earliest mediums used were fat taken from the patient's own body, and paraffin. However, both materials had disappointing results. From 1951 to 1962, various versions of a polyurethane-based sponge were experimented with, but all resulted in the breasts becoming overly firm within a year, with a 25 percent reduction in volume. Caused by capsular contracture, which occurs when the scar and fibrous tissue tightens around the implant forcing it to contract, the sponge would eventually collapse. Furthermore, this type of implant had other complications, such as multiple scars and high risks of infection.

Meanwhile, silicone was invented by the Dow Corning company during World War II, and by 1961, physicians began injecting free silicone into the breasts. However, this process resulted in a high rate of infections and skin loss. By 1963, a silicone gel implant was introduced, consisting of a dense gel surrounded by a thick shell. Anchored to the chest wall with a woven patch, the main problem with this first-generation implant was that it again caused the breasts to become too firm within a short period of time.

In 1965, an inflatable breast implant was developed by a French plastic surgeon named Arion, but was not available to the North American market until 1969. The implant consisted of a silicone or silastic shell that was implanted into the breast and then filled to the desired volume with a saline (salt water) solution. This early version of the inflatable breast implant also caused the breasts to become hard, and although the saline solution was not harmful to the body if the implant ruptured, the patient would instantly become flat-chested on the damaged side. Indeed, statistics show that as many as 76 percent of these early types of implants burst within three years. Over the next decade, improvements were made to the saline implant, and the rates of rupturing dropped significantly. Currently, the modern saline inflatable implant, which is used throughout North America, has a 10 to 15 percent chance of deflating over ten years.

In 1974, another type of implant, called the double-lumen, was invented. This consisted of an inner shell (or lumen) that was infused with a silicone gel and an outer case that was filled with saline. The theory behind the double-lumen implant was that the outer shell would protect against any silicone leakage, which was causing a problem in some patients, including local irritation of the breasts and the subsequent discovery of small pieces of silicone in the lymph nodes.

Furthermore, it allowed for adjustments in the size of the implant to be made after it had been put in place. However, although the double-lumen implant continued to be used, the extra coating did not prove to be effective against leakage.

Although some surgeons preferred the inflatable saline implants, by the mid- to late 1980s most surgeons in North America were using a newer form of silicone gel, which incorporated a thicker shell to help restrict leakage. Then in 1992, a legal case came to the attention of the media. In it, the patient claimed that her silicone implants had caused her medical harm, leading to an autoimmune disease. Although there were no scientific data to back up the claim that a ruptured silicone implant could cause diseases such as lupus, scleroderma, and arthritis, the legal case snowballed into a class action suit against implant manufacturers. Dow Corning, one of the biggest makers of implants, went into bankruptcy protection and settled. This implied guilt on their part, and the public began to believe that silicone was a major factor in the development of autoimmune diseases, resulting in a complete ban of silicone implants in the United States, Canada, and France. Although surgeons stated they found no correlation

Chapter 12| Breast Enhancements

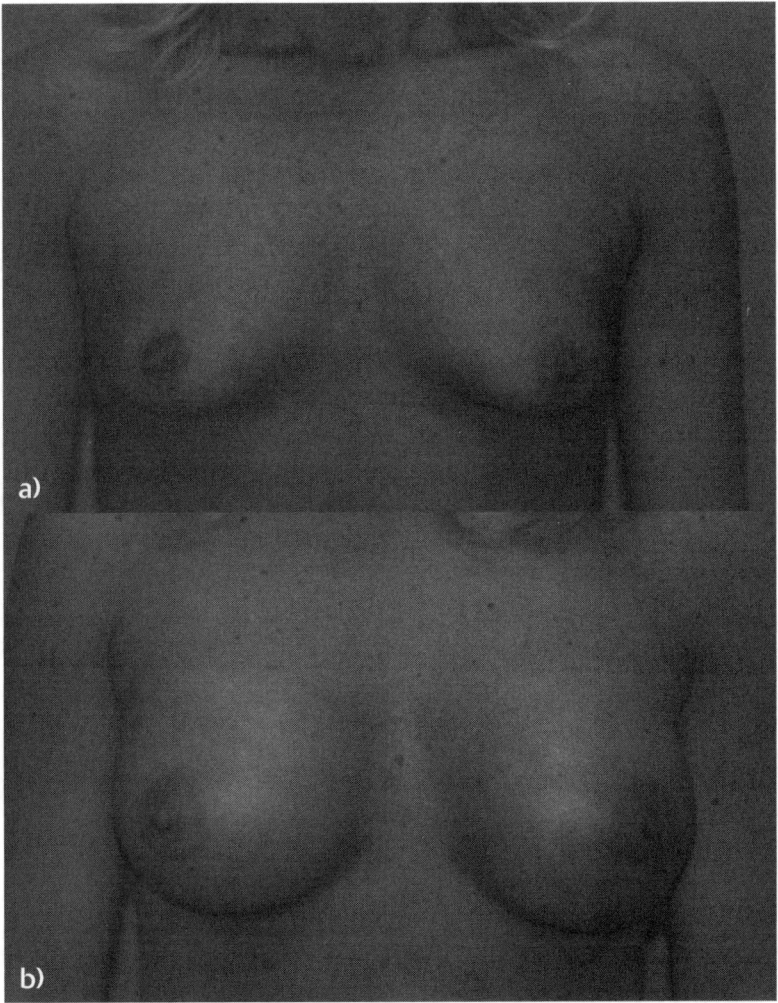

Breast augmentation with normal saline implants. a) pre b) post

between silicone and disease, and the implants continued to be used successfully in Europe with minimal complications, the ban continued in North America and France because there was a lack of information to prove that the substance did not cause a problem.

In 1994, after an extensive study conducted by the Mayo Clinic, it was found there was no relationship between silicone implants and connective tissue diseases. Yet the ban persisted.

Then in April 2000, the U.S. Food and Drug Administration (FDA) also reported there was no connection between silicone implants and autoimmune diseases, and later that year, another study was released by the U.S. National Cancer Institute that found no changed breast cancer risk connected with any version of breast implant. In November, 2001, it was reported in an issue of *Arthritis and Rheumatism* that after an extensive study, no connection had been found between silicone implants and rheumatoid arthritis. France lifted its ban, but Canada and the United States maintained their prohibition of the silicone implants. Currently, they can only be used in Canada if preoperative approval is obtained from the Ministry of Health, and in the United States, you must be enrolled in an ongoing clinical study.

Meanwhile, in 1993 a new type of silicone implant was developed in Europe called the cohesive gel implant. The silicone in it was cross-linked at the molecular level, making it even thicker, with the consistency of a gummi bear. If it was cut in half, the silicone would not leak out, thus virtually eliminating any local complications associated with silicone leakage. Soft and pliable in its texture, the cohesive gel implant gave a natural look and feel to the augmented breast, and became the implant of choice in Europe.

In September 2000, Julie Khanna was the first surgeon in Canada to augment a women's breasts using the new Inamed cohesive gel implants. Although she has to obtain special permission for each and every patient, she currently uses the Spectrum Inamed of cohesive gel implants in the majority of her patients.

If you are considering breast augmentation to increase or restore the volume of your breasts, there are a variety of implants available, and a consultation with an experienced plastic surgeon will help you decide which type is best suited to you. During this consultation, the surgeon will not only enquire about your health history, but will also determine what results you are looking for. Your natural anatomy needs to be respected, and therefore your

Chapter 12| **Breast Enhancements** 179

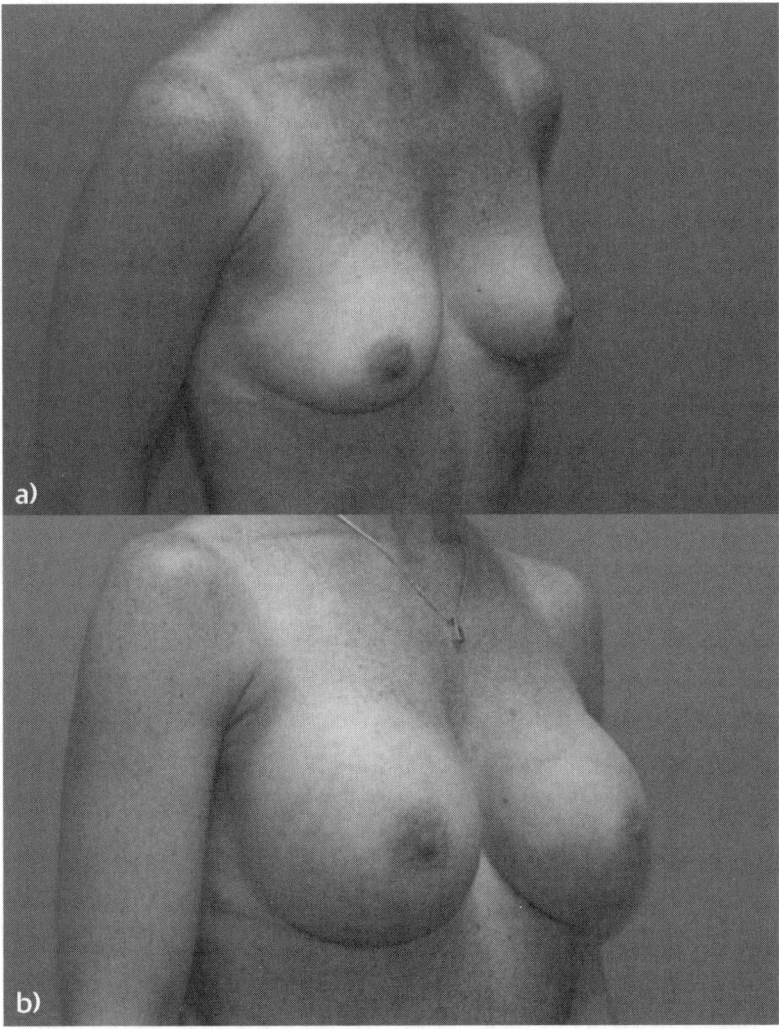

a) pre b) post augmentation with shaped cohesive gel Inamed style 410 implant.

body and breast shape and size will be taken into consideration before deciding on the implant. It is also a good idea to bring in any photographs of breasts or cleavage type that you find appealing to help the surgeon understand what you're looking for. At home try putting dry rice in a zip lock bag and put it in a unpadded bra to assess the volume of the implant you are looking for. Implants are measured in milliletres or grams but not by cup size.

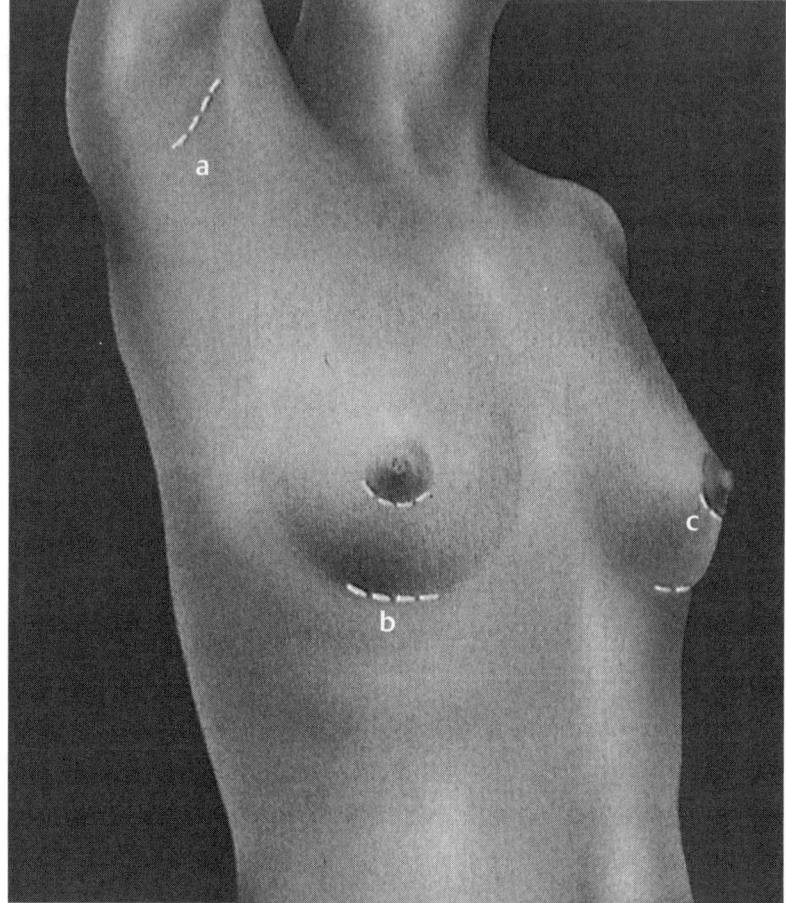

Incisions can be made: a) in the armpit b) under the breast crease or c) around the areola

Technique: For both the saline and silicone gel implants, the operations will usually be performed under a general anaesthetic in a clinic or hospital. Taking no longer than forty-five to sixty minutes to complete, you will be admitted as an outpatient. An incision will be made either under the crease of the breast, through the armpit, or around the nipple area to create a pocket where the implant will be inserted either on the top of the pectoral muscle or under it. If the implant is positioned on top, it will give you more lift and won't interfere with your pectoral muscle function. However, if the implant is

Chapter 12| Breast Enhancements

placed under the muscle, it will be better hidden, especially if you are thin. There are also less risk factors associated with the implant going under the muscle, such as capsule formation (see complications). Once the implant has been inserted, the incision will be closed, usually using absorbable sutures.

Downtime: Three to seven days.

Complications: There will be the usual risks associated with being under a general anaesthetic, and expect some soreness and discomfort for a few days after surgery. Bleeding during and after this procedure is rare, but if it does occur it may have to be drained with a needle or may require a second surgery. The greatest concern surrounding this operation is that infection may occur. Although happening in less than 1 percent of surgeries, if the implant does become infected, it will have to be removed and cannot be replaced for at least six months.

In about 20 percent of saline implants, and less than 5 percent of gel implants, you will feel and/or see a rippling effect in the skin, caused by the scalloped edge of the implant. A scar wall surrounding the implant, called the capsule, will occur without exception, and in about 20 percent of all patients the scar wall will be tender and/or hard to the touch. Capsule formation can also cause the implant to move or become distorted in shape. Inserting the implant under the muscle will drop the rate of capsule formation by about half. There is also seems to be less problem with capsule formation with cohesive gel implants.

In 10-15 percent of both saline and gel implants, rupture will occur within ten years and the implant will have to be replaced. If saline implants rupture, they will eventually go totally flat, causing an unnatural look to the breast area, while the rupture of gel implants may slightly alter their shape, causing small divots or new ripples to form. After surgery, feeling around the nipple area may be increased, decreased, or completely gone, and it can vary on each of the breasts.

There is no increased or decreased risk in breast cancer associated with any type of implant. However, they will all interfere with mammograms, so it is important that you have the mam-

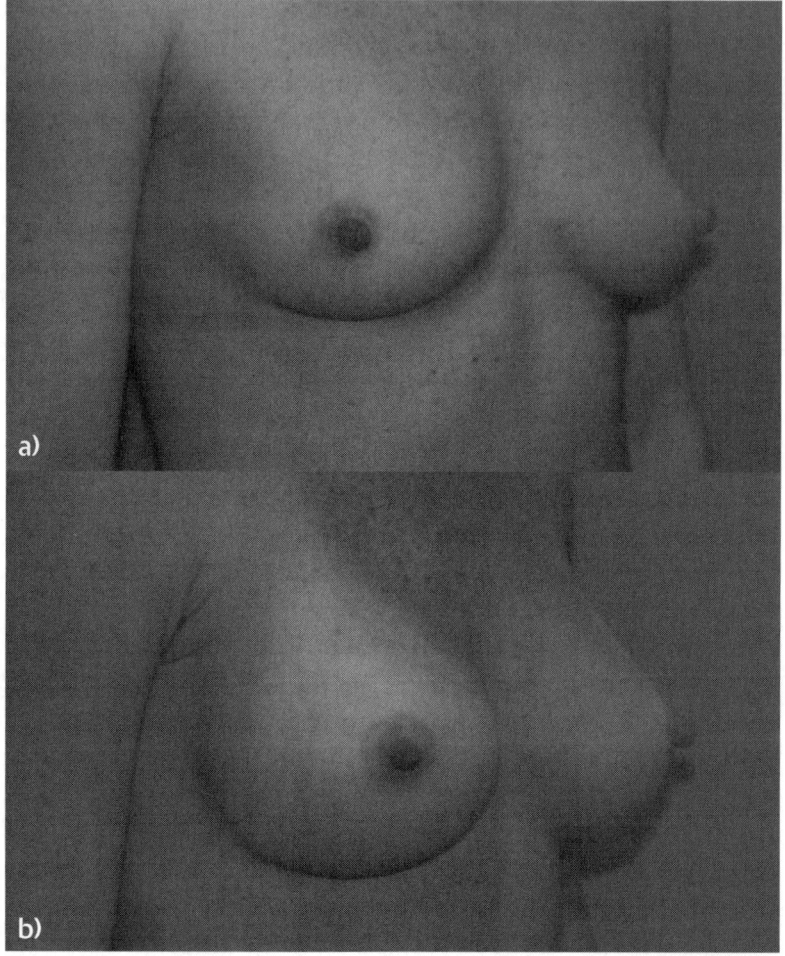

a) pre b) post augmentation with round cohesive gel Inamed style CMH (high projection implants)

mogram taken at a clinic that understands the nature of breast implants. Ask your surgeon to recommend such a facility. Assume that you will not be able to breast-feed after the procedure.

Post-treatment: Despite some claims that implants placed under the muscle will cause more pain that those positioned over the muscle, there is no significant difference in the level of discomfort that you will feel afterwards. If you are experiencing pain, a medication such as Tylenol 3 can be taken.

Chapter 12| Breast Enhancements

You may shower the day after the operation.

It is interesting to note that most patients believe the size of their breasts are too big immediately following the procedure, but after six weeks, they believe the breast size is too small. In reality, it will take up to six months before you see the final shape and volume.

Results: A breast augmentation will increase your breast size and volume. You will also get some lift to the breast.

Ideal Candidate: If are over the age of eighteen and believe your breast size is too small either because of genetics, pregnancy, breast-feeding, or weight loss, you will benefit from a saline or gel implant. Those who have had a mastectomy or have a congenital abnormality such as a difference between the size and shape of their breasts will also see their figures improved with a breast augmentation.

How Often: You must assume you will have repeat surgery at some point because of rupture, capsule formation, and changes in lifestyle. On average, surgery is done every ten years, but could occur after one, five or thirty years. If you don't have a problem, you will not need another surgery.

Cost: $6,500–$7,500 for a saline implant; $8,500–$9,500 for a cohesive gel implant.

MOST COMMONLY ASKED QUESTIONS

Question: Can I still work out after a breast augmentation?
Answer: If the implants are placed under the breast tissue, you will be able to work out at normal high intensity four to six weeks after the procedure. If they are placed under the pectoral muscle, try to avoid pure pectoral muscle exercises as they will often push the implant down and outward.

Question: Will I still get a lift when I get a breast reduction?
Answer: With a traditional breast reduction, not only is the breast size reduced but the breast is also lifted. As an added benefit, the areolar area is usually decreased in diameter at the time of surgery.

Question: Is it true that I will never be able to breast-feed if I have surgery on my breasts?
Answer: You must assume that you will be unable to breast-feed after surgery. If you are uncomfortable with this, then it is recommended that you wait until after you are done having children before proceeding with any breast surgery.
Question: I have asymmetrical breasts. Is this normal?

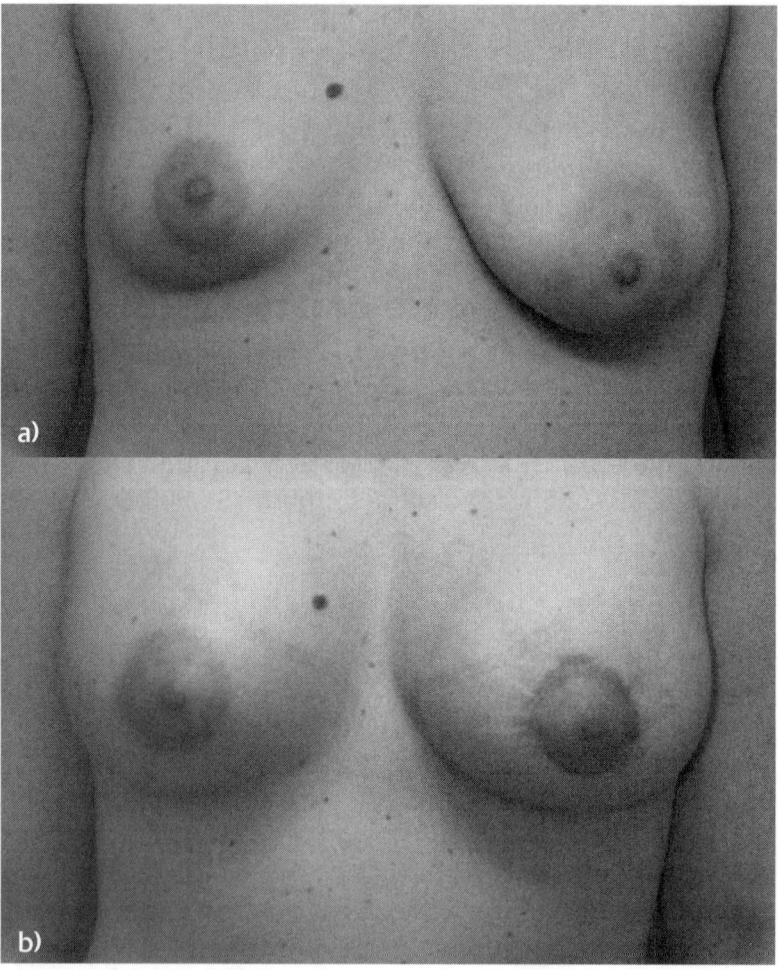

a) Asymmetry of the breasts. b) Post-bilateral augmentation with cohesive gel Inamed style 410 - shaped implants and mini lift on the left side. Two different sized implants were used.

Answer: Most women have differences between the right and left breast, and because this is sometimes not noticed by the woman before surgery, her physician will usually point it out. Breast surgery can correct these asymmetries, but small differences between the right and left breast might always exist.

Question: Are silicone breast implants safe?

Answer: After the ban of liquid silicone gel implants in 1992 in Canada, the U.S., and France, many people felt very uncomfortable with the re-introduction of silicone implants into the marketplace. It is important to understand that even in 1992, there was no solid scientific evidence demonstrating a correlation between systemic diseases such as lupus, arthritis, and scleroderma and silicone gel implants, either intact or leaked. There is, however, some correlation of local irritation of the breasts associated with leaking liquid silicone implants. Cohesive gel implants are a new "gummi-bear" type of implant that are softer and more natural feeling, but do not leak as the older silicone models have done. Furthermore, the newer liquid silicone gel is also semi-cohesive, and therefore they do not openly leak as a pure liquid might.

Question: Can breast implants ever look or feel real?

Answer: There are certain factors that will improve the likelihood of a breast implant looking very natural. If you choose a size that is proportioned to your body's shape and dimensions, the implant will look more natural, while selecting one made out of a softer substance, such as cohesive gel, will make it look and feel more natural.

Chapter 13

Cosmetic Dentistry

Aging not only plays havoc with our bodies, but also with our smiles. As our teeth become discoloured and worn over the years, it can affect the way we feel about ourselves and how others perceive us. We tend to smile less, worrying about how our teeth look, and those around us mistakenly believe we are unhappy or have a negative personality. Chipped, missing, or crooked teeth can also distort the face, and in the process, lower our self-confidence. But thanks to modern dental technology, there are a multitude of ways to brighten our smiles and our outlook on life.

While veneers, bonding, and crowns will cover discoloured and unsightly teeth, simple and noninvasive bleaching methods, performed in the dentist's office or at home, can enhance your smile and take up to five years off your face. Missing teeth can be replaced with bridges and implants, while crooked teeth can be repaired with a combination of orthodontic work and cosmetic dentistry.

The options are many, but first and foremost, you must see a qualified specialist to discuss what procedure would best suit your individual needs. But because cosmetic dentistry is not taught in dental school and there is no structured or governing body to regulate the industry, it can be difficult to find a true expert in the field. In fact, any dentists can call themselves a specialist in cosmetic dental procedures, but in reality, it takes many courses, learning, and years of experience before a dentist is a true authority on the subject.

During your initial consultation with the cosmetic dentist, he or she will go over your complete medical history and will give you a full dental examination. X-rays may or may not be taken, and any problems such as untreated cavities or gum disease will have to be addressed before cosmetic treatments can begin.

WHITENING
Bleaching Gels

Background: There are several ways to whiten and brighten the teeth at home using a bleaching gel. Although manufacturers would have you believe that toothpaste alone will produce a sparkling smile, there is usually not enough strength in the product to achieve any satisfying results. However, there are certain types of stain removers that come in the form of a toothpaste, that will somewhat lighten the stains caused by red wine, coffee, tea, and tobacco. You can also purchase bleaching kits, which involve either painting your teeth with a whitener, using a tray filled with a gel, or covering your upper and lower teeth with a strip saturated with a whitening substance. Compared to a professional system that uses 16 to 24 percent of the bleaching gel (which is made up of hydrogen or carbamide peroxide that transforms into oxygen molecules to break up the stains in the tooth enamel), these "over-the-counter" methods typically have only a 6 percent value, and although they can work well for some people, usually they are not strong enough to provide dramatic results.

Chapter 13| Cosmetic Dentistry

Professional bleaching gel systems involve using various strengths of the hydrogen or carbamide peroxide in a tray that has been specifically designed for your mouth, and will be used at home under the supervision of the dentist.

Technique: During the initial appointment, the dentist will take an impression of your teeth, so that a mouth tray can be formed. The fitted tray will ensure that the bleaching materials, which will be inserted into the tray, do not come in contact with your gums. When ready, you will take this tray home along with a bleaching gel and instructions on how to wear it. Depending on the severity of staining, you may be asked to use the system overnight, for a half day, or for an hour in the morning and another hour at night, for a period between one and two weeks.

If you have particularly sensitive teeth (which can occur if you have a tendency to brush across your gum line, rather than up and down, causing small nicks to form), you may want to ask your dentist for a fluoride gel that can be inserted in the tray and worn for about an hour before you begin bleaching.

Downtime: None.

Complications: Your teeth may be sensitive for up to two weeks afterwards.

Post-treatment: Your dentist may want to see you to check on your progression while your at-home treatment is underway. After the bleaching process has been completed, you should avoid any staining foods, drinks, or tobacco for at least a week.

Results: Your teeth will be four to seven shades lighter than their original colour.

Ideal Candidate: The bleaching gels work quickest and best on those who have yellow to slightly brown stains on their teeth. If you have dark brown to greyish teeth, which is sometimes caused by taking medication such as Tetracycline while your permanent teeth are still developing, this system can take from one to six months to produce results.

How Often: Once. Depending on your lifestyle, the whitening effects can last for up to two years.
Cost: $400–$600 per treatment.

Light Source with Gel (Zoom)
Background: Usually performed with an arc light, the Zoom technique (which is a trade name) involves coating the teeth with a gel solution that typically consists of hydrogen peroxide and then "hitting" the teeth with a high-intensity light source. Although the system has received wide media attention because it is the procedure most often used on extreme makeover television shows, it can provide disappointing results.
Technique: Done in the dentist's office, and taking no longer than one to one and a half hours, a protective substance will be coated over your gums and mouth. A bleaching gel will be applied to your teeth, which will then be hit by a light source, causing the teeth to instantly change colour.
Downtime: None.
Complications: There is a high rate of sensitivity after this procedure; however, it will subside over a period of time. Twenty to 40 percent of patients do not get the desired results and will require further treatment.
Post-treatment: Avoid staining foods, drinks, and tobacco for at least a week after the procedure.
Results: Your teeth will be four to seven shades whiter than their original colour. However, several treatments may be required to obtain these results.
Ideal Candidate: If you have yellow to slightly brown stained teeth, you may benefit from this procedure. Dark brown to greyish teeth will most likely require several treatments in order to achieve the desired results. This may also be a good procedure to consider if you have a single discoloured tooth.
How Often: Once or more initially, depending on the desired results. The whitening effect will last for up to two years.
Cost: $800 per session.

Laser with Gel

Background: Utilizing a laser that acts on its own or activates a gel substance that has been applied to the teeth, this method of whitening achieves instantaneous and satisfying results. However, the laser often causes high sensitivity in the teeth for a prolonged period of time.

Technique: Taking approximately an hour to complete, the dentist will cover your gums and lips with a protective coating. Depending on the type of laser used, a bleaching gel may or may not be applied to your teeth. When this has been completed, your teeth will then be hit by the laser.

Downtime: None.

Complications: Your teeth may become extremely sensitive after treatment and the discomfort can last for a prolonged period of time.

Post Treatment: Avoid any staining foods, drinks, and tobacco for at least a week after the procedure.

Results: Your teeth will be four to seven shades whiter than their original colour.

Ideal Candidate: If you do not have overly sensitive teeth to begin with, and have yellow to slightly brown stains, the laser whitening technique will be of benefit. If your teeth are dark brown to a greyish colour, or if you have sensitive teeth, you should consider another type of procedure. This technique is also a good choice for lightening a single discoloured tooth.

How Often: Once. Depending on your lifestyle, the whitening effect can last for up to two years.

Cost: $800–$1,500 per session.

TOOTH RESHAPING

Background: If you have a chipped tooth, or teeth that are otherwise healthy but only slightly out of alignment, tooth reshaping is considered to be a very effective way to correct the problems. Utilizing a variety of rubber wheels, disks, and drills to recontour the tooth without removing a great deal of enamel, the method is fast and virtually painless.

Technique: Depending on the number of teeth to be reshaped, the procedure will take only a minimal amount of time and may or may not require a local anaesthetic. Using various instruments, the dentist will reshape or round off the tooth, and then polish it.
Downtime: None.
Complications: If too much enamel or tooth structure is removed, it may leave the tooth open to decay.
Post-treatment: None.
Results: This procedure will correct chipped or slightly misaligned teeth.
Ideal Candidate: If you are considering veneers because you have chipped or slightly misaligned teeth, you should consider this procedure first.
How Often: Once.
Cost: $300–$450 per session.

DENTAL BONDING

Background: By building up layers of acrylic resin to the front of the teeth, a cosmetic dentist is able to reshape and change the colour of the tooth through dental bonding. Giving the illusion of straighter, whiter teeth, the procedure is also an easy way to replace old amalgam (silver) fillings. However, dental bonding is time-consuming and because the acrylic substance is not strong, it will easily chip, necessitating in a repair that will involve stripping the entire tooth and beginning again. Furthermore, the bonding material doesn't last long and tends to fade and discolour over time.
Technique: Usually performed under a local anaesthetic, the tooth or teeth are prepared with a drill, as the dentist attempts to do as little damage as possible to the enamel. Then the teeth will be treated with an acidic solution that allows the acrylic resin to adhere to the natural tooth structure. The resin will then be applied in layers to the front of the tooth. Depending on the amount of work to be done, the procedure can take from one to two hours to complete.

Chapter 13| Cosmetic Dentistry

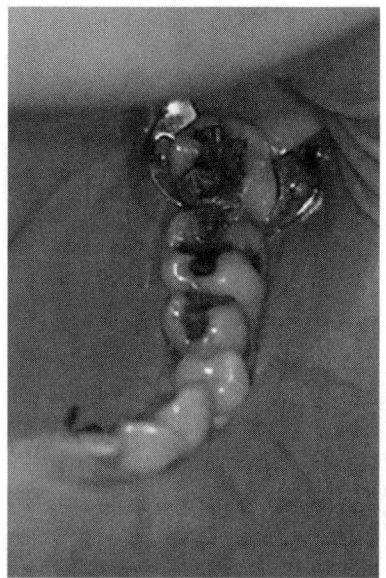 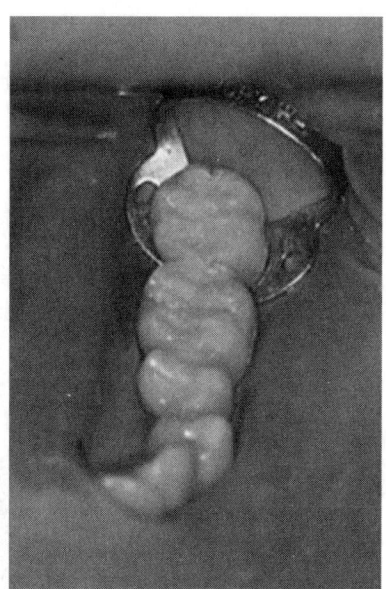

Replacing old amalgams with resin bonded fillings.

Downtime: None.
Complications: The acrylic resin tends to fade and discolour over time. It will also chip easily, requiring a second procedure to be done. Decay can occur underneath the bonding.
Post-treatment: Avoid staining foods, drink, and tobacco for at least a week.
Results: Dental bonding will correct minor gaps, chips, and cracks in the enamel, as well as giving the illusion of whiter teeth. It will also replace old, silver fillings.
Ideal Candidate: If you have discoloration on your teeth and minor imperfections or noticeable silver fillings, you may benefit from this procedure.
How Often: Once. Results can last from three to five years.
Cost: $400 per tooth.

PORCELAIN VENEERS

Background: Similar to bonding in its application, but using a substance that is much harder and many times more resistant to fracture, porcelain veneers are a popular choice for those

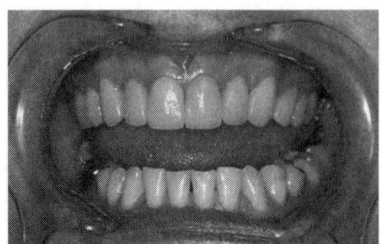 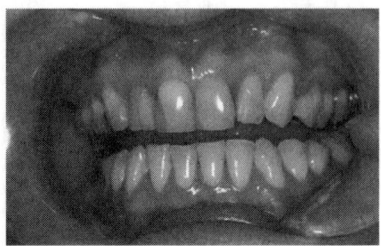

Ten veneers to lengthen and brighten discoloured teeth.

who have discoloured teeth with various imperfections. Because the porcelain has the ability to recreate the subtle nuances of translucency and contour of the enamel, the procedure gives a natural looking and long-lasting result. The application of the veneers is most often performed after gum re-contouring and bleaching of the surrounding teeth.

Technique: In your initial visit, the teeth will be prepared for the veneers by using a drill, usually done under a local anaesthetic, with the dentist being cautious to do as little damage to the tooth structure as possible. Then an impression of your teeth will be taken, and temporary veneers will loosely be applied with spot bonding to each individual tooth. You will then make a second visit to the dentist, who will remove the temporaries and bond the permanent veneers to the tooth.

Downtime: None.

Complications: There may be some sensitivity to the gums and teeth, which should not last for more than twenty-four to forty-eight hours. Decay can occur underneath the veneers.

Post-treatment: None.

Results: Porcelain veneers will make your teeth look whiter and straighter.

Ideal Candidate: If you have discoloured teeth that have imperfections or are misaligned, you are a good candidate for veneers.

How Often: Once. Veneers can last from ten to fifteen years before they need to be replaced.

Cost: $800–$1,500 per tooth.

CROWNS

Background: Used to treat teeth that have undergone root canal work, or have sustained large fillings, crowns involve removing the entire surface of the tooth and replacing it with a cap-like structure. Although the colour of the crown can initially be matched to the surrounding area of teeth, it will not usually change colour with time, as your natural teeth will. Furthermore, if your gums recede, a dark line may form at the base of the crown.

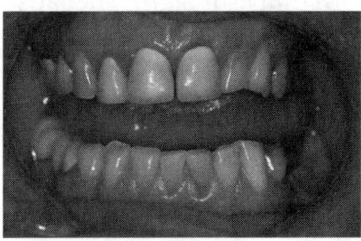
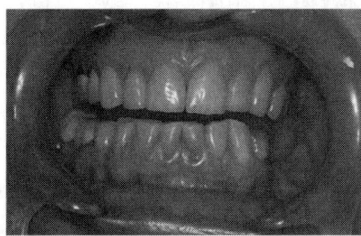

Five porcelain veneers and three porcelain crowns. This person had just recently finished having implants in the lower left and plans to veneer the lower anteriors.

Technique: Requiring two sessions with the dentist, the initial work will usually be done under a local anaesthetic and will involve the removal of 1.5 to 2 millimetres of tooth structure. An impression will then be taken of the prepared tooth and sent to a laboratory, where a porcelain crown will be fabricated. During the waiting period for the permanent crown, which is approximately one to two weeks, a temporary crown made of acrylic will be worn.

In the second visit, the porcelain crown will be adhered to the original tooth, covering the entire structure to just under the gum line. If bite is a problem, the crown will be fused to a semi-precious metal to give added fracture resistance to the forces of the bite.

Downtime: None.

Complications: There may be some discomfort or pain for a short period of time following the procedure. The colour of the crown is permanent and over time, may not match the surrounding colour of teeth. If the gum line recedes, a dark, unsightly line will form at the base of the crown. It is also possible for the crown to fracture, and decay can occur underneath.

Post-treatment: A medication such as Tylenol may be taken for any short-term pain. Avoid chewing on the area for at least two hours.

Results: The crown will cover a tooth that has sustained damage from root canal work or large fillings, matching it up to the surrounding teeth.

Ideal Candidate: If you have a tooth that is unsightly because of damage from previous dental work, and it will not sustain a porcelain veneer, you are a definite candidate for a crown.

How Often: Once. A crown should last from ten to fifteen years.

Cost: $800–$1,000 per tooth.

BRIDGES

Background: When a tooth is missing between otherwise healthy teeth, the space can be filled by a tooth replica or bridge. Applied in much the same way as a crown, the difference with a bridge is that three connecting crowns will be fabricated and placed over the existing teeth and space. The downside to this technique is that the healthy teeth on either side of the gap will have a substantial amount of tooth structure removed in order to prepare the bridge.

Technique: Requiring two visits, the initial session will be done under a local anaesthetic. The dentist will first prepare the two existing teeth on either side of the space by removing some of the tooth structure. An impression of the area will be taken and sent to a laboratory, where a permanent bridge will be fabricated within one to two weeks. In the meantime, a temporary will be applied. During the second visit, the temporary bridge will be removed and the permanent will be inserted. This will be done by fitting an end of the bridge over one of the existing teeth, while the other end of the bridge is fitted over the tooth on the opposite side of

Chapter 13| **Cosmetic Dentistry** 197

the gap. When in place, the bridge spans tooth, space, and tooth by way of three crowns set as a distinct unit.
Downtime: None.
Complications: There may be some discomfort and pain following the procedure that can last for twenty-four to forty-eight hours. Because the porcelain bridge will not discolour, there may be some variances in colour with the surrounding teeth over time. If the gum line recedes, a dark line can form at the base of the bridge. It is possible for the bridge to fracture, and decay can occur underneath.
Post-treatment: A medication such as Tylenol can be taken to alleviate any pain or discomfort.
Results: Gaps and spaces caused by missing teeth will be filled.
Ideal Candidate: If you have lost a tooth, you are a good candidate for this procedure.
How Often: Once. A bridge should last from ten to fifteen years.
Cost: $2,200–$3,000.

IMPLANTS
Background: Made up of titanium alloy, an implant is an artificial root that binds to surrounding bone on a microscopic level. Acting on its own as an anchor for a porcelain crown or bridge, the insertion of the implant to replace a missing tooth causes no harm tto the adjacent healthy teeth. Lasting up to thirty years or longer, these implants are fast becoming the preferred choice of dentists when correcting spaces caused by missing teeth.
Technique: Performed under a local anaesthetic by a dental surgeon, and taking from one and a half to two hours to complete, the procedure involves a hole being made in the bone at the site of the missing tooth, into which the implant will be screwed. The skin will then be closed with sutures.

It takes approximately three to six months for the surrounding bone to adhere to the surface of the implant (called osseointegration), and form a root replica. Then you will return to the dentist's office to have an impression made of the site. This impression will then be sent to a laboratory, which will fabricate the crown or bridge that will be attached to the implant approximately two weeks later during a subsequent procedure.

Downtime: One to two days (following the initial session).

Complications: There will be swelling and tenderness that can persist for up to ten days after the initial procedure. There is also a risk of infection. Smokers and diabetics are especially prone to prolonged healing periods. There is less than a 5 percent chance that the implant may be rejected.

Post-treatment: Following your initial surgery, pain medication such as Tylenol can be taken. Do not take any acetylsalicylic acid products such as Aspirin. Your dental surgeon may also advise you to rinse with a peroxide solution.

Results: An implant will allow a crown or bridge to be inserted to cover any spaces or gaps, without compromising other healthy teeth.

Ideal Candidate: If you have missing teeth, the implant procedure can be of benefit to you.

How Often: Once. An implant can last for thirty years or longer.

Cost: $1,200–$2,600 per tooth.

MOST COMMONLY ASKED QUESTIONS

Question: Will whitening my teeth hurt?

Answer: Approximately 30 percent of all patients experience some temporary sensitivity during and following the procedure. In almost all cases this can be controlled by taking a medication such as Tylenol.

Question: How long can I expect the whitening effects to last?

Answer: Your teeth will stay white for approximately twelve to twenty-four months, depending on your eating and drinking habits. A "touch-up" kit can restore the whiteness in twenty-four to seventy-two hours.

Question: Will my veneers look natural?

Answer: Although some patients opt for the "Hollywood" white picket fence look, most prefer a more subtle smile, which means straighter and somewhat whiter teeth. Ultimately, it is up to you to tell the dentist what you want.

Question: How long will my veneers last and do I have to be careful with them?

Answer: Well-done veneers should last a minimum of five years, with the typical lifespan being ten to fifteen years. Veneers are extremely durable and the only care required is good brushing and flossing to maintain the gum tissue surrounding the veneer and prevent decay from entering the body of the tooth behind the veneer.

Question: Why should I consider an implant to replace a missing tooth, when a bridge or crown would do?

Answer: The first criterion for tooth replacement and bite restoration is to perform the least invasive procedures possible. Although the jawbone will be entered with a foreign object (titanium implant) in order to perform an implant, it keeps from removing the tooth structure of two of the other teeth in order to replace a single tooth. With the predictability and high success rate of implants, this procedure is considered to be the most efficient way to replace a missing tooth.

Chapter 14

Hair
Restoration

A full head of healthy, shining hair may be a woman's crowning glory, but if she is losing her once beautiful tresses, it can be a major source of frustration and embarrassment. Most common in men, hair loss can begin in our late teens and slowly progress as we get older. Fortunately for the fairer sex, unless caused by stress or medical problems, hair loss in women tends to result in an overall subtle thinning, as opposed to the full and very noticeable baldness that many men endure. In the past, our only options were to cover the thinning hair with a wig or hairpiece, wear a different type of hair style in an attempt to camouflage the loss, or try prescription drugs that had to be taken or topically applied over a long period of time, and worked to a limited degree. We certainly never gave much thought to hair transplants. That procedure was only for men ... or so we believed.

Restorative hair surgery is an extremely underutilized treatment for women. Indeed, studies show that 95 percent of all people receiving hair transplants are men. In fact, this method of correcting baldness caused by androgenetic alopecia (hair loss caused by a combination of inheritance from one or both of your parents, along with hormonal effects) is the leading cosmetic procedure for the male population, followed by Botox injections and liposuction.

While hair transplants will work well for people with a genetic condition, it is not a procedure to be considered for hair loss that is induced by medication, such as chemotherapy, or a major stressful event such a divorce, death in the family, loss of a job, a serious illness that has required hospitalization, or even the loss of a great deal of weight. Called telogen effluvium, this type of hair loss is temporary and will generally reverse itself after a period of time. Probably the most commonly seen telogen effluvium occurs in women who have given birth. A few months after delivering the baby, they will often begin to notice large clumps of hair falling out. It is apparent on their shoulders, pillows, and in the shower. Caused by synchronization of hair follicles, the shedding typically continues for a few months before it spontaneously reverses itself without any treatment.

Another type of hair loss (called alopecia areata), which cannot be treated with transplants, is often identified by its patchy appearance. There is a genetic predisposition to alopecia areata, as shown by the fact that it sometimes runs in families, and may also be associated with other medical problems such as thyroid disease, vitiligo (loss of skin pigment resulting in white patches), or vitamin B12 deficiency. These associated conditions will require medical therapy, should they be discovered during routine laboratory testing for the cause of the alopecia.

If you are considering hair restoration surgery, you must first consult with a specialist in the field, who will go over your medical history in depth. If you have various active diseases such as discoid lupus or lichen planopilaris, which may cause patchy scalp hair loss, scalp rashes, and scarring that can destroy transplanted hair follicles, you may not be a suitable candidate for this procedure. Persons who have bleeding disorders may also be turned down for hair restoration surgery, since an abundance of tiny cuts will be made in the scalp in which the hairs will be transplanted. If there is profuse bleeding during the surgery, it may cause the transplants to dislodge and the hair won't grow.

During this initial consultation, the doctor will also determine when your hair loss began, the rate at which it is occurring, and whether your hair is shedding (which is usually caused by telogen effluvium) or losing its density. This history, combined with a physical examination, will determine what type of hair loss is taking place and whether or not it can be treated with hair transplants. Typically, androgenetic alopecia hair loss slowly worsens over the years. Therefore, it is important for an eighteen-year-old who is losing his or her hair to realize that transplants may not provide good long-term results, since the hair loss will be ongoing. Gains that are made initially through hair restoration surgery may be less evident as further hair loss occurs naturally over time. Although controversial, some physicians believe that it is best to wait until later in life before proceeding with such surgery.

During the consultation, the physician will also look at the quality and colour of your hair. The less contrast there is between skin and hair colour, the better the results. For example, someone with an olive-toned complexion with blonde or grey hair that has a curly or wavy texture, will have significantly better results than the person with black, straight hair and a pale complexion. Curly hair gives a false impression of thicker density, while blonde or grey hair matches the scalp colour better than darker hair, thus providing improved camouflage of the balding scalp.

Because there is so much to take into consideration before deciding on whether or not you want to proceed with hair restoration, it is extremely important that you develop an honest and frank rapport with your specialist. The doctor must know your expectations beforehand, and let you know whether or not they can be met. It is also vital to see someone who is qualified to perform this procedure. As with all other types of cosmetic treatments, there is no governing body to regulate this field and anyone in the medical profession can call themselves a "hair restoration specialist" by simply taking a weekend course. Mistakes made by an unskilled person may or may not be correctable, so ensure that your doctor is well-trained in hair transplant surgery.

Background: The idea that hair could be transplanted was first documented in Germany in 1822. And although attempts were made at hair transplanting in the 1930s, it wasn't until 1959 that Norman Orentreich was credited with originating hair restoration for male pattern baldness. Discovering that hair always takes on the characteristics from the site in which it is taken, Orentreich was able to remove hair from either the back or side of the head and transplant it to the balding area using a punch grafting technique. This method, which remained popular for several years, involved using a biopsy tool that punched out small pieces of skin with hair attached to it, and moving it to a less dense site by creating more punch holes and dropping the piece of tissue in. However, the resulting look was often less than satisfactory as the patient's scalp took on a "doll's head" look, with several clumps of hair growing in the otherwise balding spots. Eventually refinements were made to the technique, whereby the punch holes became smaller. Then surgeons began to look at the advantages of taking strips of skin rather than circles, and by the early 1990s, a new procedure was developed using the strip method, which is now considered to be standard.

Further refinements permitted more natural-looking transplants. Because hair grows in units (called follicular units), it was realized that by harvesting one or more of these groupings and transplanting them together, instead of randomly taking different hairs, the resulting growth pattern would appear more natural. This method of follicular unit grafting is now universally accepted as the most efficient way to transplant hair.

Technique: Before the day of the surgery, you will be given a series of blood tests to ensure there are no underlying medical problems, which could compromise the transplant results or endanger you should the surgery proceed. You will also be asked to keep your hair at the donor site (where the hair will be taken from, usually at the back or sides) at least 4 or 5 centimetres long, to help hide the scar. For two weeks prior to surgery, you must not take any blood-thinning medication, particularly acetylsalicylic acid (ASA). For a week prior, you should also avoid certain anti-inflammatories, such as ibuprofen, as well as vitamin E and alcohol. You may or may not be given a prescription for an antibiotic to be taken the day before surgery, and you will be given a prescription for pain medication such as Tylenol 3, Percocet, or Demerol, which you may require during the surgery and for a few days afterwards.

On the day of surgery, you will have your blood pressure checked and be given a medication such as Valium to relax. Photographs will be taken and then markings will be made on your head to ensure the transplants will look natural with a hairline that is age appropriate. A local anaesthetic will then be administered to the donor site. Although the needles are fine, expect some discomfort during this procedure. After the area is frozen, the surgeon will cut a strip of skin that is variable in length, but can run from ear to ear, and anywhere from 6 to 10 millimetres in width. The surgeon will either cut this strip as a single intact unit or, by using a multibladed scalpel, take two to four strips of skin at once. The donor site is then cleansed, and if there is any bleeding, the areas will be lightly cauterized, taking care not to damage other existing follicles. When this initial stage of the procedure is completed, which takes approximately thirty minutes, the incisions will be closed with sutures or staples.

You will then be able to rest for one to two hours. During this time, technicians will prepare the grafts by cutting the strips into tiny pieces that will have anywhere from one to

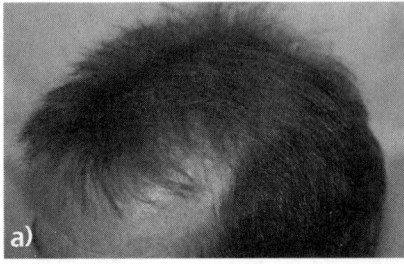 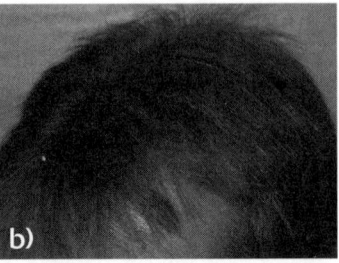

a) *Before* hair transplantation, there is prominent receding of the hairline at the temples; additionally, the scalp hair is sparse, creating a 'see-through' appearance.
b) *After* hair transplantation, the hair density is markedly improved. The receding hairline was maintained to create an age-appropriate appearance. Moving the hairline too far forward is generally thought to appear unnatural in the presence of significant balding.

four hairs per unit. During preparation, the tissue is stored in a moist solution to ensure its viability.

When this procedure is finished, the recipient site (where the hairs are being transplanted) is then prepared by administering a local anaesthetic, and adrenaline to help reduce bleeding. Using a needle or needle-like device, the surgeon will then poke tiny holes into the area, or if the grafts have more hair per follicular unit, he or she may cut slits or slots with a surgical blade in which the tissue can slide. It is very important that the surgeon makes these openings at the same angle that the existing hair is growing so that the transplants match the natural growth pattern. Also, the smallest follicular units will be placed at the front, closest to the forehead, while the hairs with a thicker diameter will be positioned behind to give a denser look.

Taking between one to three hours to perform, depending on how much hair is being transplanted and whether or not there is any bleeding, the actual insertion of the follicular units will usually be made by a nurse and a trained assistant, who will also check on each transplant. When the procedure is finished, the surgeon will perform the final check before a lubricating medication or antibiotic ointment is applied to both sites, which are then covered with a nonstick dressing. Most often, the head will then be wrapped in a turban-like

Chapter 14| **Hair Restoration** 207

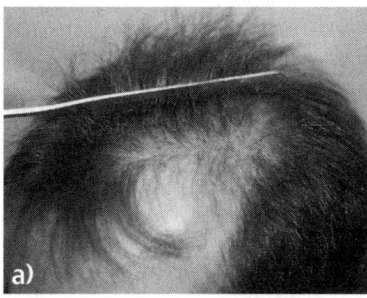 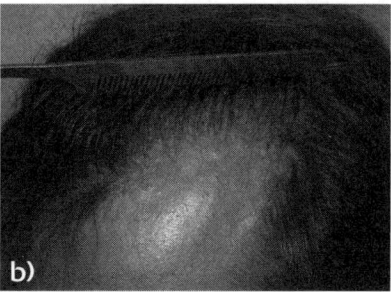

a) Close up of the left frontal scalp *before* hair transplantation.
b) Close up of the same area *after* hair transplantation. Note that the hairline appears very natural. Use of small follicular grafts insures that there is no 'clumping' of hair follicles. The increased hair density is clearly apparent.

bandage. If the head is not wrapped, the patient will have to remain in the office for one to two hours to ensure there is no bleeding.

Downtime: Two to seven days.

Complications: Although marked bleeding is very uncommon, it may occur. Expect some pain and swelling on the forehead, sometimes extending to the eyelids, that can last for a few days afterwards. There is also an extremely rare chance of infection, which occurs in less than 1 percent of patients. Because nerves may have been severed during the procedure, expect some itching for a few days. You may also have an alteration of sensation on the scalp, which can be permanent, but sometimes subsides within one to two years. In very rare cases, a piece of the scalp can become black and crusted then die (called scalp necrosis). And after the procedure, you will experience a temporary period of hair loss (called post-surgical effluvia), caused by the shock of the surgery. While scarring at the recipient site is minimal, scarring will occur at the donor site and, in 10 to 15 percent of patients, can result in a raised red (hypertrophic) scar. Approximately 10 percent of the transplants will not take.

Post-treatment: You may take the prescribed medication for any pain (see above), but do not ingest any products containing acetylsalicylic acids, such as Aspirin. On the day following the surgery, you will return to the doctor to have the bandage removed. After forty-eight hours you may cleanse the donor area by soaking your head in the bathtub for ten to fifteen minutes and then gently massaging to loosen any crusts that have formed. To cleanse and soften the transplanted site, soak the area twice a day with a wet cloth and then apply a lubricant such as Vaseline to keep the area moist. After a couple of days, you may gently comb through the area, taking caution not to dislodge the grafts.

Results: Although the hair will look stable for a few weeks, it may then begin to shed and look worse in the area that has been transplanted. However, in three to eight months, you will begin to see significant growth that should look natural and denser than prior to the transplant.

Ideal Candidate: If you have significant hair loss due to androgenetic alopecia, with good hair density in the potential donor area, and your hair colour is blonde or grey and curly in texture, you will most likely have excellent results from this procedure. If your hair is very dark and your complexion is pale, you will still get good results, but they will not be as significant as the individual with blonde or grey hair.

How Often: This will depend on how bald you are and the amount of thickness you desire. If you are completely bald on the top of your head, a single session in which a few thousand hairs are transplanted will result in a sparse look, and further sessions will be required. If your hair is thinning, a single session may be sufficient, although you may wish to have further transplants as your natural hair diminishes with age.

Cost: $2,500–$10,000 per session. (A reasonable estimate for a session in which 2,000–3,000 hairs are transplanted will be between $6,000 and $7,000. Individuals satisfied with a smaller session will pay less. The cost of subsequent sessions varies with the amount of grafts needed or desired.)

MOST COMMONLY ASKED QUESTIONS

Question: What is hair transplantation?
Answer: Hair transplantation refers to the surgical movement of permanent hair with its roots to an area of bald or balding skin. Hair transplantation is an effective and permanent solution for certain types of hair loss.

Question: How long does the procedure take?
Answer: This is an office procedure and the duration varies with the number of grafts being transplanted. Typically, a session may last from three to six hours.

Question: Will it look natural afterwards?
Answer: In the hands of a well-trained and experienced physician, and using the newer techniques with smaller grafts, the hair will grow in the proper direction with a feathered hairline and a highly aesthetic result.

Question: Will I treat the transplanted area like the rest of my hair?
Answer: The hair is your own, and just like all of your other hair, it will grow, can be washed, curled, shampooed, permed, and styled as desired. Once the transplants are completed, no special maintenance is required.

Question: Will there be a scar?
Answer: The site from where the hair is taken is usually left with a fine scar line that is hidden by the permanent hair in that area. Rarely, one may see thicker or wider scars. There will also initially be some tiny marks where the grafts have been placed, but they will not be easily seen after two to four months.

Question: Can women benefit from a hair transplant?
Answer: Women with localized thinning on the top of their heads or thinning around the temples are often good candidates for hair transplant surgery. It is important to first discuss your thinning hair with a physician who is well-versed in hair loss, such as a dermatologist and/or an endocrinologist, to ensure there are no other treatable reasons for your hair loss.

Chapter 15

Choosing
a Qualified Specialist

Selecting a reputable, experienced professional who has been thoroughly trained in performing cosmetic procedures or surgery is the single most important factor in determining the success of your treatment. This can be difficult because there isn't any college or university designation to imply that someone truly is a specialist in the cosmetic field. Furthermore, because there is no governing body to regulate who can call themselves a "cosmetic specialist," the term can be used by any medical doctor, who may or may not have had training or special qualifications on the procedure that they are claiming to be their expertise. Because of this, cosmetic surgery has now been over run by general practitioners, aestheticians, dentists, and others. Unfortunately, these nonspecialists performing aesthetic procedures are usually limited to offering one or two procedures that they may have learned how to perform, often over a week or a weekend course.

When you are considering a cosmetic procedure, it is important to see a dermatologist or a plastic surgeon, who will be familiar with a wide range of surgical and nonsurgical options, which they can offer to their patients. You will also want to ensure that your plastic surgeon is certified by either the American Board of Plastic Surgery in the United States or by the Royal College of Physicians and Surgeons of Canada. If you are seeing a dermatologist, you will want him or her to be certified by the American Board of Dermatology or the Royal College of Physicians and Surgeons of Canada. In both countries, this certification means that the surgeon or dermatologist has completed all the required training and passed all exams. It also implies that these physicians have proven themselves to their peers and colleagues and demonstrated an eagerness to attain and maintain level of quality in their chosen profession. However, in the United States, you must be cautious if someone calls themselves "board eligible." This will mean that the physician has completed his or her training but has not gone on to take the necessary examinations.

When choosing a surgeon, it is also wise to select someone who is a member of the American or Canadian Society for Aesthetic Plastic Surgery or the American Dermatological Association or the Canadian Dermatology Association. A general membership in these organizations denotes an ongoing interest in aesthetic plastic surgery and dermatology and a commitment to maintaining credentials by continual education in this field.

You may wonder why it is so vital to have your procedure done by someone who can almost be considered overqualified. If a problem develops during your cosmetic surgery or procedure, which can happen, could that specialist deal with it if he or she hasn't been extremely well-trained in most aesthetic procedures? A well-rounded specialist, also has the further experience and education that provides them with a breadth of knowledge beyond the here and now, they will be able to deal with any unpredictable situation that can happen during the surgery or procedure. Not only are they trained to complete the operation or procedure, but also to deal with any complications that may arise.

Chapter 15| Choosing a Qualified Specialist

It is also important to see a specialist who offers a full spectrum of care and surgical procedures. If you are concerned about your abdomen, for instance, and consult with a doctor who only knows how to perform liposuction, he or she may not recommend that you actually require a tummy tuck, since they don't know how to perform such a procedure. And during any consultation, don't be afraid to ask questions about the doctor's credentials. No qualified surgeon or dermatologist will balk at your inquiries. If they do, you should continue your search for the right doctor. If you're uncomfortable asking the physician these types of questions, ask their staff to show you the doctor's certificates. And don't just look at them—read them. Although the certificate may look impressive, it may just mean the physician has taken a weekend course on the subject. Pre- and post-operative photographs of other patients should also be available to you, along with testimonials. If you want to speak to another patient who has had the same procedure done that you are considering, this should also be an option. Above all, you should never feel intimidated, rushed, or pressured while trying to gather information about your doctor and the procedure you are contemplating.

If the surgery or procedure is going to be performed at a clinic as opposed to a hospital, you should know whether or not it is an accredited facility. Although accreditation is currently not mandatory in Canada and in several states in the U.S., having your procedure performed in an accredited facility will ensure that there is a commitment to a certain standard and level of care that your surgeon wants to deliver to you. Done on a volunteer basis, the doctor is paying to have the facilities checked by either the American or Canadian Association for Accreditation of Ambulatory Surgery Facilities. This means the facility established emergency protocols and is appropriately equipped to deal with emergency situations. Even if the clinic is accredited, ensure that if the operation is being done under a general anesthetic, there will be a board certified or Royal College certified anaesthesiologist present. Furthermore, make certain your surgeon has privileges at a local hospital. That will tell you the surgeon have passed the credentials committee at that hospital, and if there are circumstances that come up during the operation there is someplace to take you.

Finally, it is crucial to the success of your operation that you find a specialist you are comfortable talking to. You want someone who listens and understands your needs. Developing a good rapport with your doctor, and thoroughly discussing your expectations, means there is far less of a chance that you will be dissatisfied with the results. An affable relationship with your doctor will also come into play after your surgery or procedure, when you may become anxious about your recovery, or have questions that may not have been addressed prior to the surgery. Knowing that your physician is accessible to you to meet your needs during this time will offer an extra level of comfort.

To begin the process of selecting a qualified specialist, you should first ask your general practitioner to recommend a surgeon or dermatologist who specializes in cosmetic procedures. You may also want to talk to other people you know who have undergone aesthetic treatments and obtain referrals from them. Books, magazine articles, and the Internet are other sources of helpful information. If you are using the Internet, you can go to the websites of the various affiliations and organizations listed at the end of this book to obtain the name of a cosmetic specialist in your locality or to ascertain if their facilities are accredited.

This is your face, your body, and, potentially, your life that you are putting into the hands of someone else. Do your homework, ask the questions, and take however long you want before making any decisions. So if you've completed your research and are still not comfortable with having a certain procedure done, don't do it. And while it is true that the clock can be set back by the variety of surgeries and procedures we've discussed in this book, true timeless beauty—the type that shines from the eyes of an eighty-five-year-old woman who has never had a touch of cosmetic surgery in her life—comes from within.

Chapter 16

Preparing for Your Surgery

Once you have decided to go ahead with a procedure or surgery, it is very important that you prepare yourself in order to help your team of specialists give you the best results possible. Following is a general guideline of what you can do to ensure your treatment is a success.

DIET AND EXERCISE

You always want to be in the best physical shape that you can be before proceeding with any surgical intervention. A healthy diet and regular exercise will help maintain a weight that is appropriate for your body size and shape. This will help assist in defining the areas that may require more surgical attention in liposuction, an abdominoplasty, or breast surgery. It will also decrease your risk of having problems such as clotting and other surgical complications. A regular exercise program will also mean that not only will you be walking into the surgery or procedure healthy, but you will more quickly return to an active lifestyle after the surgery.

Radical and fanatic dieting should be avoided prior to any procedure. Anything that causes a significant imbalance in your body can interfere with proper wound healing, which requires increased energy, vitamins, and minerals. Therefore, make certain to maintain a well-balanced diet prior to any surgical procedure. Remember, surgery is not a replacement for good health and exercise.

WATER
Drinking extra water for several days prior to a general anaesthetic will make you well hydrated going into the surgery, and can decrease post-operative nausea and complications.

SMOKING
Smoking is detrimental to any procedure, causing small blood vessels to go into spasm every time a cigarette is lit. Over time this is part of the difficulties that smokers have with circulation. When you have any type of surgery, your body relies on these small blood vessels to supply blood to the area and help it heal. Therefore, if you can quit smoking six weeks prior to the operation and six weeks afterwards, this will significantly help in the wound healing process, since 50 percent of the initial healing occurs within six weeks. Other complications such as pneumonia and increased risk of infection are also associated with smoking and can undermine your final result.

Smoking is also a significant contributor to aging. Among other things, it will cause lines to form around your mouth from puckering, and will also result in a loss of elasticity and collagen. Because smoking speeds up the aging process, you may lose the results that were obtained with any cosmetic procedure.

MEDICATIONS
Medications that cause blood thinning should be avoided for at least a week prior to surgery. These include over-the-counter medications such as Aspirin and anti-inflammatories

Chapter 16| **Preparing for Your Surgery**

such as Advil and Aleve. Vitamin E should also not be taken. Make sure you speak with your surgeon or physician about all medications and over-the-counter products that you are taking, including any herbal remedies, since many of these are also associated with bleeding and interference with wound healing.

Birth control pills and hormone replacement medication should also be stopped for a period of time to be determined by your physician before and after major surgery because of the increased risk of deep vein thrombosis. If you are pregnant, you should avoid cosmetic procedures and surgery.

MEDICAL HISTORY
Discussing your medical history in depth with your physician or surgeon, prior to your procedure or surgery is an important part of the overall process. Furthermore, informing your surgeon and your anasthesiologist about any family history regarding nausea after surgery, and the details of your previous surgeries, can help prevent problems.

ATTITUDE
Going into surgery with a positive mental attitude, with a full understanding of both the surgical procedure and the postoperative care involved will make your recovery much easier. Being well prepared and informed can only result in you feeling much more comfortable about your upcoming treatment.

WHO TO CONTACT FOR FURTHER INFORMATION

In Canada:

The Royal College of Physicians and Surgeons of Canada
774 Echo Dr.
Ottawa, ON
K1S 5N8
613-730-8177
www.rcpsc.medical.org

The Canadian Society for Aesthetic Plastic Surgery
2334 Heska Rd.
Pickering, ON
L1V 2P9
www.csaps.ca

The Canadian Dermatology Association
1385 Bank Street, Suite 425
Ottawa, ON
K1H 8N4
613-738-1748
www.dermatology.ca

The Canadian Association for Accreditation of Ambulatory Surgery Facilities
2334 Heska Rd.
Pickering, ON
L1V 2P9
905-831-5804
www.caaasf.org

Chapter 16| **Preparing for Your Surgery** 221

In the United States:

The American Board of Plastic Surgery
Seven Penn Center, Suite 400
1635 Market St.
Philidelphia, PA
19103-2204
215-587-9322
www.abplsurg.org

The American Board of Dermatology
Henry Ford Health System
1 Ford Place
Detroit, MI
48202-3450
313-874-1088
www.abderm.org

The American Society for Aesthetic Plastic Surgery
ASAPS Central Office
11081 Winners Circle
Los Alamitos, CA
90720
800-364-2147
www.surgery.org

The American Association for Accreditation of Ambulatory Surgery Facilities
5101 Washington St., Suite 2F
Gurnee, IL
60031
888-545-5222
www.aaaasf.org

Index

A

abdominoplasty. *See* tummy tucks
ablative resurfacing techniques
    chemical peels, 54–58, 60
    dermabrasion, 58–59
Accutane, 28
acne, 17, 28, 31, 50
    Blu-U therapy and, 39–40
    nonablative lasers and, 41
    TCA peels and, 54
acne scars
    dermabrasion and, 59
    laser techniques and, 77–80
    microdermabrasion and, 33
    nonablative lasers and, 40–42
    superficial chemical peels and, 35–36
    TCA peels and, 55
age spots. *See* brown/age spots
aging, 9–28
    extrinsic, 10
    four main events of, 31
    intrinsic, 9–10
    genetics and, 9
    societal attitudes toward, 3–4
all-trans retinoic acid, 17. *See also* retinol
aloe vera, 22
alopecia, androgenetic, 202, 203. *See also* hair loss; hair restoration
alopecia areata, 202. *See also* hair loss; hair restoration
alpha hydroxy acids (AHAs), 6, 20–21, 27, 54
alpha lipoic acid, 23
alpha tocopherol, 20
American Association for Accreditation of Ambulatory Surgery Facilities, 213, 221
American Board of Dermatology, 212, 221
American Board of Plastic Surgery, 212, 221

American Dermatological Association, 212
American Society for Aesthetic
    Plastic Surgery, 5, 6, 144, 162, 221
amino acids, 23, 25, 149
aminolevulinic acid (ALA), 36
antioxidants, 10, 19, 23–25
Argireline, 22
Arjerolin. *See* Argereline
arm lift, medial, 162–64
Artecoll, 4, 93–94, 100

B

bariatric surgery, 168
beta hydroxy acids (BHAs), 21–22
blepharoplasty. *See* eyelid lifts
Blu-U therapy, 28, 39–40
Botox, 4, 5, 6, 7, 8, 22, 31, 84, 88,
    96–99, 100, 102, 109, 116, 202
brachioplasty. *See* arm lifts, medial
breast enhancement surgery, 169–85
    asymmetry and, 174, 185
    augmentation, 175–83
    breast cancer and, 174, 181
    breast-feeding and, 174,
        182, 184
    exercise and, 183
    mammograms and, 182
    reduction, 170–74
    risks and complications, 181–82
    types of, 169–70
broken blood vessels, 30, 50, 66–70, 81, 83
brow lifts, 115–118, 124
brown/age spots, 11, 12, 17, 30, 31,
    34, 36, 38, 40, 50, 53, 62,
    laser techniques and, 70–73
buttock enhancement surgery, 165–67

C

Canadian Association for
    Accreditation of Ambulatory
    Surgery Facilities, 213, 220
Canadian Society for Aesthetic
    (Plastic) Surgery, 212, 220
capsule formation (in breast), 181
carbon dioxide lasers, 6, 60, 63–66,
    78–79, 84
Carruthers, Jean, 96
cheek augmentation, 127–30
    implants and, 128–29
cheiloplasty, 89
chemical peels
    medium to deep, 54–58
    superficial, 34–36
chin reshaping, 130–33
coenzyme Q10, 23
cold sores. *See* herpes simplex
collagen, bovine, 88, 89
collagen cosmetic products, 23
collagen treatments, 88-90
continuous wave lasers, 70–72
CoolGlide laser, 76, 81
CoolTouch laser, 40
copper, 23
"cosmeceuticals," 26
cosmetic dentistry, 187–99. *See also*
    teeth; teeth whitening
cosmetic procedures
    men and, 7
    popularity of, 5–7
    patient expectations and, 7–8
    spending on, 5
cosmetic products, 15–28
    physician-marketed, 28

Index

"cosmetic specialists," 211
CosmoDerm, 88
CosmoPlast, 88

D

deep vein thrombosis (DVT), 158, 160, 165, 219
dental procedures. *See* teeth; teeth whitening
dermabrasion, 32, 58–59, 60
DermaDeep, 93
DermaLive, 93, 100
dermatologists, certification of, 212
dimethylaminoethanol. *See* DMAE
diode lasers, 75–76
DMAE, 24
Dow Corning company, 175, 176

E

ear surgery, 136–37, 140
Einstein, Albert, 61
ELOS technology, 37
Erbium laser, 66, 78, 84
Excimer laser, 77
exfoliant products, 32
eyelid lifts, 118–22, 124

F

facelifts, 110–115
    after other procedures, 122–23
    endoscopic, 111, 112
    risks and complications, 111, 113
    smoking and, 123–24

facial contouring, 126–140
    cheek augmentation, 127–30
    chin reshaping, 130–33
    ear surgery, 136–37, 140
    nose reshaping, 133–36
fat transplantation, 95–96
Featherlift technique, 48–50
FeatherTouch laser treatment, 63
fillers, temporary vs. permanent, 100
Fitzpatrick skin type classification, 14
FotoFacial RF, 37
Fractional Photothermolysis. *See* Fraxel laser treatment
Fraxel laser treatment, 42–44, 51
free radicals, 10, 11, 19

G

GentleLASE laser, 75
Glogau Classification system, 12–13
glycolic acid, 20, 34
glycolic acid peel, 50
grape seed extract, 24
green tea, 24

H

hair, ingrown, 85
hair loss, 118, 201–03, 207
hair removal, 75–76, 83
hair restoration surgery, 7, 201–09
    patient suitability for, 202–04
    history of, 204–05
    preparation for, 205
    risks and complications, 207
    women and, 201–02, 209
hair transplantation. *See* hair

restoration surgery
herbal supplements, 101–02
herpes simplex, 33, 35, 38, 59
hyaluronic acids, 24–25, 30, 90–93
Hylaform, 90

I

implants, cohesive gel, 178, 185
implants, dental 197–98, 199
implants, double-lumen, 176
implants, silicone
    autoimmune diseases and, 176–78, 185
    ban on, 176–78, 185
    in breast, 175–78
    breast cancer risk and, 178
    in buttocks, 166–67
    facial, 128–29, 139,
    use in Canada, 178
intense pulse light (IPL) facials. *See* photo facials

J

Jessner's peel, 34, 35, 60
Juvederm, 90

K

Klein, Jeffrey, 143
Kojic acid peel, 34, 36, 60

L

L-ascorbic acid. *See* vitamin C
lactic acid, 20

laser therapy, 61–84. *See also* specific brand names
    carbon dioxide, 63–66, 78–79
    continuous wave, 70–72
    endovenous, 82, 84
    Erbium, 66, 78–79
    history of, 61–62
    long-pulse YAG, 70, 75–76, 81
    nonablative, 40–42
    pulsed dye (PDL), 66–70, 76–78, 80–81
    Q-switched, 72–74
leg veins, spider vs. varicose, 103
leg vein treatments, 81, 82, 84, 103–08
Levulan, 28, 36–37, 38, 50, 51, 83
LightSheer laser, 76
lip augmentation, 89
liposuction, 141–149, 150–51
    arm lifts and, 162–63
    breast reduction and, 172
    buttock enhancement and, 166
    cheek augmentation and, 128–29
    external ultrasound-assisted (EUAL) method, 144
    facelifts and, 112
    fat transplantation and, 95
    history of, 142–44
    large-volume, 146
    popularity of, 5, 7
    risks and complications, 146–47
    traditional method, 142–43
    tumescent method, 143, 144–6
    tummy tucks and, 155, 168
    ultrasonic method, 142, 144
    weight loss and, 150
long-pulsed Alexandrite lasers, 75
long-pulsed Ruby lasers, 72, 73, 83
"love handles," 144, 149

Index

M

mammoplasty, reduction. *See* breast enhancement surgery, reduction
mammoplasty, augmentation. *See* breast enhancement surgery, augmentation
mastopexy. *See* breast enhancement surgery, breast lift
matrixil, 25
Mayo Clinic, 177
melasma, 60
men, cosmetic surgery and, 7
mentoplasty. *See* chin reshaping
mesotherapy, 149–50
microdermabrasion, 4, 5, 6, 7, 31–34, 50
moisturizers, 16–17, 20

N

National Cancer Institute, 178
N-Lite System lasers, 40
nonablative resurfacing techniques, 29–51
nonsurgical procedures, growth of, 6–7,
nose reshaping, 133–36
    closed vs. open rhinoplasty, 134
    to alter ethnic appearance, 140

O

oglio-peptide, 25
olive oil, 25
Orentreich, Norman, 204
otoplasty, 136–39

P

Pan G "facelift ," 48
peptides, 26
Perlane, 90
phenol peel, 34, 56–58
phlebectomy, ambulatory,107
photo facials (IPL facials), 36–39, 50, 51, 83
photo-aging, 11–13, 17
physician-marketed cosmetic products, 28
plastic surgeons
    certification of, 212
    choosing of, 211–15
plastic surgery clinics, accreditation of, 213
pigmentation, changes in, 20, 30. *See also* photo-aging
pregnancy, 18, 28, 60, 103, 219
    tummy tucks and, 161, 167
proanthocyanidin, 24
profiloplasty, 126
pulsed dye laser (PDL) treatment
    short pulse, 66–68
    long pulse, 68–70, 76–78

Q

Q-switched lasers, 72–74, 83

R

Radiothermoplasty, 44. *See also* thermoplastic contouring
Renova, 6, 17, 19
Restylane, 4, 5, 90, 91, 93, 100, 101

Retin-A, 6, 17, 19, 54
retinol, 17, 18, 19
retinyl palmitate, 18, 19
rosacea, 62, 68, 69, 83
Royal College of Physicians and Surgeons of Canada, 212, 220
rhinoplasty. *See* nose reshaping
rhytidectomy. *See* facelifts

S

"saddlebags," 149
salicylic acids, 21. *See also* beta hydroxy acids
scars
    keloid, 80–81
    acne, 77–80
Sciton laser, 76, 81
sclerotherapy, 84, 104–06, 108
SilkTouch laser, 63
skin
    aging of, 4, 9–16
    purpose of, 29
    three layers of, 29
    types of, 13–14
skin cancer, 13
soy, 26
smoking, 218
Smoothbeam laser, 40, 42, 79–80, 84
stretch marks, 76–77, 84
Sulamanidze, Marlen, 48
sun damage. *See* photo-aging
sun protection factor (SPF), 14, 15, 27
sunscreens, 14–15, 16, 27
surgical body-lifting techniques, 153–68. *See also* specific techniques

T

tanning, 13
tattoos, 4, 73–74, 83
TCA peel. *See* trichloracetic acid peel
teeth
    bonding and, 192–93
    bridges and, 196–97
    crowns and, 195–96
    implants and, 197–98, 199
    porcelain veneers and, 193–94, 199
    reshaping of, 191–92
teeth whitening, 188–91, 198
    by bleaching gels, 188–90
    by light source with gel, 190
    by laser with gel, 191
telogen effluvium, 202, 203
ThermaCool, 44
ThermaLift, 44
Thermage, 31, 44–48, 50–51, 60, 79, 84, 109, 122
thermoplastic contouring, 44–48
thigh lift, 164–65
tocopherol acetate, 20
tocotrienol, 20
torricelum, 26
tretinoin, 17–18
trichloracetic acid (TCA) peel, 54, 60
tummy tucks, 154–62, 167
    in combination with other surgeries, 156, 168
    history of, 154
    liposuction and, 155, 168
    obesity and, 161
    pregnancy and, 161, 167–68
    risks and complications, 158, 160
    types of, 155

Index

U

Ubiquinone, 23
UltraPulse laser, 63
U.S. Food and Drug Administration, 178

V

varicose veins, 82, 103, 104–06
Vbeam laser, 68, 77
vein stripping, 106–07
vitamin A, 17, 27, 84. *See also* retinol, tretinoin
vitamin C, 19, 27
vitamin E, 20, 24
vitamin K, 26
V-Star laser, 68, 77

W

Wise geometrical pattern, 171
wrinkles, 87–102
    Artecoll for, 93
    Botox for, 96–99, 100
    causes of 30, 87-88
    collagen treatments for, 88–90
    cosmetic products for, 17–27
    fat transplantation for, 95–96
    hyaluronic acids for, 90–93
    laser therapy for, 63–66
    photo-aging and, 11–13
    Vitamin A and, 17

Y

YAG laser, 70, 75–76, 81, 83

Z

Zocchi, Dr. Michael, 144
Zoom whitening technique, 190
Zyplast, 88
Zyderm, 88